MORE PRAISE FOR *THE TUNNEL*

"This beautifully written book is a powerful and moving story of a family's struggle with mental illness and the turmoil and love that were involved. It's a necessary book that can help us all to better understand mental illness and how to deal with challenges and grief."

—**Walter Isaacson**, bestselling biographer of *Steve Jobs, Benjamin Franklin, Albert Einstein* and *Elon Musk.*

"As diagnostic terms go, "mental illness" can be too tidy, too gentle. Full-blown psychosis deals a savage blow — perhaps especially to a privileged family expecting the very best from life. Tripp Friedler's book is an act of courage. He somehow found it in himself to lucidly detail a beloved and promising son's descent into catastrophe. Anyone whose life has been touched in this way will admire *The Tunnel* and learn from it."

—**Jed Horne**, Pulitzer Prize-winning journalist and author of *Desire Street* and *Breach of Faith*

"Run to your nearest bookstore and get this gripping account of a family who displays amazing grace under pressure. And pray you are never tested as they were."

—**Randy Fertel**, author Winging It: *Improv's Power and Peril in the Time of Trump, The Gorilla Man and the Empress of Steak: A New Orleans Family Memoir*

"A moving and remarkable account of a how mental illness impacts the entire family. While the Friedler family's experience is not uncommon, their story is told in a way that grips the reader and provides unique insights into what families have to go through as they watch their young adult child descend into psychosis, struggle to get the correct diagnosis and engage with a mostly dysfunctional treatment system. This is a must read for any family dealing with the mental illness of a loved one."

—**Andrew Sperling**, former Director of Legislative Advocacy, National Alliance on Mental Illness (NAMI)

"*The Tunnel* in many things at once: a devastating account of bipolar disorder in a young man's life, an honest reckoning with the limitations of parental care, and an urgent call for deeper empathy in our educational, policing, and carceral institutions. This book will stay with me."

—**Stéphane Gerson**, author of *Disaster Falls: A Family Story*

"This moving testament to a son feels like a necessity—to Tripp Friedler, who had the bravery to write it with such eloquent honesty, to the hard task of drawing life lessons from the memory of the son who was so deeply loved, and to any reader who has faced the hardest puzzles life as a family can offer.

—**Fred Schruers,** author of *Billy Joel: The Definitive Biography*

the tunnel

A MEMOIR

TRIPP FRIEDLER

Trost Publishing
New Orleans, LA.

Copyright 2024 By Tripp Friedler
All rights reserved.
First edition 2024

Printed in Canada

Image credits
first picture David Halliday
end picture: Heidi Friedler

Cover art by Pat McGuiness
Book layout by *the*BookDesigners

All people, locations, events, and situations are portrayed to the best of the author's memory. While all of the events described are true, some names and details have been changed to protect the privacy of the people involved.

ISBN 979-8-218-34242-5
ISBN (eBook) 979-8-218-34243-2

Library of Congress Control Number: 2024932011

Library of Congress Cataloging-in-Publication Data:
Friedler, Tripp
The Tunnel, a memoir
Mental Health
Bipolar Disorder
Memoir

TABLE OF CONTENTS

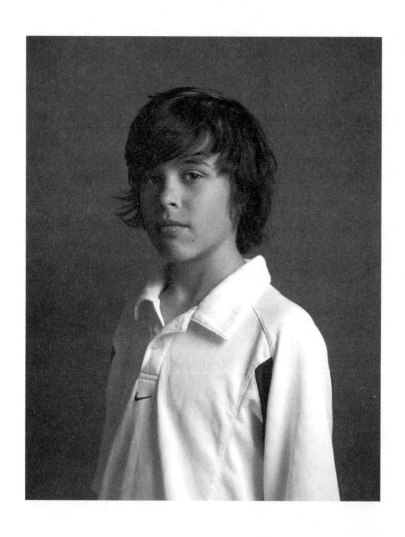

prologue

I will never forget the night Henry called from the Mississippi River Bridge. He was twenty years old, and he was crying. It was a Saturday evening in New Orleans around 6:30 p.m. on March 15, 2014. I was getting ready to go to a business dinner. My wife, Heidi, was next to me in the bedroom.

"Dad," he said in a small voice when I answered his call, "I'm scared."

"Where are you, Henry?" I replied, rattled by his tone.

"I'm parked on the side of the Mississippi River Bridge. I got out of my car and looked over. I was going to jump. I just couldn't do it. I got back in the car. I don't want to die." His voice was shaking.

"You're in the car now?" I asked, equally shaken. All I could think about was that enormous bridge and my little boy on it, looking over its edge. That sweet kid and his huge smile. The ten-year-old Henry, running around our yard without a care in the world. Not my troubled twenty-year-old, two hundred feet above a dark and murky river. Cars flying past. All these thoughts and more raced through me like an electric jolt.

"Yeah. I'm scared. I want to come home," Henry said, his voice almost a whisper. "I took a bunch of Klonopin and thought I would jump, but, when I got to the top and looked over, I couldn't do it."

We had installed a tracker on Henry's phone a few months earlier when his depression had worsened. I checked the map on my phone, hoping that he wasn't on the bridge. Hoping somehow that this was just some weird game he was playing. It wasn't. I saw the flashing blue dot in the middle of the bridge, as it blinked over the water, a cruel reminder that this was no game. All I could hear was the sound of my heart trying to escape my chest.

"Start the car and come home," I begged him. "I'm going to stay with you until you get home."

"I'm facing away from home," he said, his voice sounding a little less panicked.

"Drive over the bridge, get off at the McArthur exit, and make a turn to come home," I said like a human MapQuest except that my voice was not sweet and calm. "Have you started moving?"

"Yeah, I'm across the bridge now and making the turn to come back," he replied softly.

But I was still with him on that bridge. And all I could see was my son, alone, scared, staring twenty stories down, thinking about ending his life. Would he have panicked if a policeman or some passerby had seen his car parked in the middle of the bridge? Things could have turned out very differently. Instead, I was telling him to get off on Tchoupitoulas. To stay on it until he got home. While the easiest route home, the irony was not lost on me: Tchoupitoulas runs along the very river he had almost jumped into. Instead of floating downriver, he was now traveling upriver, toward home.

Although I knew exactly where he was because of my tracker, I would still ask just to hear his voice. I needed to know he was still with me. Other than answering my questions as to his location, he was silent. It was a fifteen-minute ride home but felt a lot longer. I heard the car pull into the driveway, and Heidi and I went downstairs to the door, our lives upended yet again.

Henry was a good-looking kid. He was just under six feet tall, with long and thick chestnut brown hair, handsome brown eyes, and an athletic build with wide shoulders. Yet, when he walked through the door that Saturday evening, he was different. He was wearing an old t-shirt and baggy shorts, both of which looked two sizes too big on him. His eyes were red and bloodshot. His hair was uncombed and unkempt, shooting out in all different directions as if trying to come off his head. He came straight up to me and hugged me, then his mom, crying and shaking. Then he said he wanted to go up to his room to sleep. He asked if I would come with him. I told him I would. Seeing Heidi's expression, I knew we needed to talk. I told Henry I would be right up. As he trudged up the stairs, Heidi's eyes followed him, then looked back at me. She had thousands of questions. I had no answers. I had a broken Henry waiting for me in his room. I knew Heidi and I needed to talk, but we both agreed Henry came first. She went to our bedroom to wait. I imagined how confused she felt and how hard it was to let me go

tend to Henry. She was his mother, and they had a close relationship. Those thirty minutes when I was with Henry in his
room must have felt like days. But she let me go, a tribute to
her patience, her trust in me, and her love for her son.

When I came into Henry's room, the lights were off.
Henry was fully dressed and under the covers. I took off my
shoes and crawled in bed with him where I held him tightly. I
had never imagined that he would attempt suicide. This was a
whole new set of circumstances, and I had trouble processing
it. I just held Henry, as if that alone could protect him from a
world that was overwhelming him. And I held him because *I*
needed it. I needed that old connection. I needed to hold him
like I had when he was a child. I needed to love him with all
my soul, thinking that might take away his pain. We didn't
talk. We laid there in silence intertwined like the branches
of a tree. After about ten minutes, Henry's breath became
shallower, and he drifted off to sleep. As I looked at Henry, at
peace and asleep, I felt small and insignificant. Seeing him so
peaceful only made his pain harder to bear. I was wide awake.
My son had almost died. A barrier and moments away from
jumping into a cold and muddy river. Why had I not noticed
the pain he was in? How could I be so dense? How was I going
to fix this one? What about Heidi? Alone in our bedroom,
worried sick about her baby boy. I had no answers. I was in
way over my head.

After about ten minutes, I moved his head gently from my
arm and quietly got up. I knew Heidi and a battery of questions

awaited me. I left Henry's room, closing the door quietly so as not to wake him, and headed to our bedroom to talk to Heidi, wondering what I would say to her. What could I say? How do you tell your wife she almost lost her son?

chapter 1

CHILDHOOD

Henry Frank Friedler was born early in the evening on April 3, 1993. It was a Saturday, and it was smack in the middle of the second game of a double header for the NCAA Men's Final Four Basketball Championship, which was in New Orleans that year. Michigan was playing Kansas in the Superdome, five miles away, but might as well have been a thousand. We were in a pretty corner room, and the sun had just set. A misty New Orleans evening light was streaming into a hospital room that felt more like a suite in a five-star hotel. The bed was in one corner, and there were chairs and a couch around a large TV on the far side of the room. The place was bigger than my first apartment.

The doctor and I were basketball fans, so we had the game on. We were a good distance from Heidi with the sound down very low. Not low enough, it turned out. "Will you two turn that off? Really? You're watching a basketball game!" she yelled between contractions. Heidi was not a basketball fan in the best of times, and these were not the best of times. Her pain was palatable. Needless to say, the TV went off.

Why she was attempting a natural birth with Henry was a simple error in judgment. She had gotten an epidural when our older daughter, Patricia Trost Friedler, was born three years earlier. Patti, clearly ready to escape, was born thirty minutes after reaching the hospital. The epidural hadn't had time to fully work. And, after Patti's birth, Heidi suffered stomach issues. So, she thought she'd try to have Henry without any drugs. We'd been wrong, and now Heidi was paying the price. Her pain was so intense she was screaming at the nurses like an old drill sergeant, which you have to understand *is so* not Heidi. At this point, the pain had won, and we were calling an audible. The doctor gave her a morphine drip to take the edge off. After that, the pain resided, and she could relax. Henry came ten minutes later.

When the doctor said it was a boy, I smiled. We didn't know that this would be a boy, though Heidi suspected as much after one ultrasound. I held him, and love washed over me like warm water. My son. My little me. Our newest addition. When babies are born, you count their fingers and toes, you make sure they are breathing well, and you are so relieved when you're told you have a healthy baby. Little did we know of the journey ahead. The fight yet to be fought.

When we brought Henry home, Patti, who was three, was enthralled. For the first few weeks, she couldn't get enough of her new baby brother. But she quickly grew bored. Henry, though, was infatuated with her. He looked at Patti like a puppy needing attention, constantly following her every move. But Patti was over her new toy, and blew him off like a high school senior would a freshman.

While Patti had been a thumb sucker, Henry was a pacifier man. Patti sucked on her thumb constantly, and luckily for her, that thumb went everywhere with her. Henry, never wanting to be without a pacifier, would always have extras. He'd have one in his mouth and one in each hand. He wore a smile that never seemed to leave his face, gooing at everyone. He was an easy baby and slept through the night by three months. He was perfect to us. We were content with our little family of four.

I was busy with work, and Heidi was busy juggling two kids and developing her interior design business. Two kids under four are not easy. Add a husband who is trying to build a business, working sixty hours a week, and Heidi's job got considerably harder. She kept us together and made life livable, though I'm sure I was not as appreciative as I could have been. Patti was in preschool, leaving only Henry at home during the week. Weekends were the tough times. I used to work Saturday mornings, meeting my dad downtown to go over our business. By the time I came home, Heidi would be frazzled and left the two kids with me—a job I was ill-equipped to handle. We went in search of weekend activities. We joined a local swimming pool, and I would take the kids there on Saturdays and Sundays to give Heidi the time she needed. We became members of the Audubon Zoo and spent afternoons there. We started our tradition of Sunday morning breakfasts at the Bluebird, our favorite local breakfast place, giving Heidi time to sleep in. The days dragged on, but the months flew by.

One night in early December, after we had put the kids down for the night, Heidi came into the bedroom. She was crying. "I'm pregnant," she announced between sobs.

I sat on the edge of the bed, like she had spoken to me in Greek. "What? How is that possible?" I asked. "We have a baby. Are you sure?"

She looked at me as if I had two heads. "Yes, I'm sure," she said, her voice rising a pitch. "This is my third test. I can't believe this is happening."

To say we were stunned would be an understatement. How could we be having another baby already? We just had Henry. Heidi was still breastfeeding, and we thought we had our birth control under control. Clearly, we were wrong. We were woefully unprepared for another child. We were still just getting used to Henry and the family we had. The thought of adding another child into the mix was overwhelming. We sat on the bed in our bedroom in silence. We had always wanted three kids, and while we would have preferred more months between them, here we were. After the initial shock wore off, it morphed into excitement. But it was an excitement that only we knew, because for the next two months we told no one. Not even our parents. We hid our secret until Heidi's clothes could hide it no more.

Since we would soon be a family of five, we needed a bigger house. Heidi had always wanted to design and build a home, and this was our chance. We put our house on the market and bought a lot in English Turn on the West Bank of New

Orleans. Building began immediately. We were expecting to stay in our Uptown house until the new one was built, but our agent found us a buyer right away. The offer was too good to pass up, so we accepted it and moved into a tiny two-bedroom apartment near Audubon Park to wait for our new house to be finished and our newest Friedler to be born.

Katherine Hackley Friedler was born on July 6, 1994. We brought her home into our tiny temporary apartment. Henry was fifteen months old at this point, and he was enthralled to have his own live baby doll. He could already climb out of his crib—the kid was athletic pretty much from birth—and had taken to walking at an early age. One Saturday, after putting him down for a nap, I went into the den to watch a football game on TV. I was in my usual prone position on the couch when I saw Henry's head peek in through the open door. He had escaped and was on the prowl. He would do this often when he was left alone in the crib, determined to be a part of whatever was going on behind his back. This usually involved Kate, and he would toddle over whenever he saw her, wanting to hold her or give Kate her bottle. He loved to cuddle, walking over to Heidi or me to crawl into our laps and hug us.

Henry wasn't our only kid who loved his pacifiers. So did Kate. And while Henry was enchanted with his little sister, this didn't stop him from climbing into her crib to steal her pacifiers. We would often find him with a pacifier in his mouth and one in each hand plus a few extra spread out amongst his toys. Sure enough, we would discover that Kate had none. The game was on!

In those early years, Heidi once visited an astrologist. This was not something either one of us was really into, but a friend convinced her to go. The woman plied Heidi with questions. "Do you have twins?" she asked. Heidi said no, and the woman looked confused. "Do you have kids very close in age?" she asked again. Obviously, the answer to this was yes. "Well, then you do have twins. They are energy twins." The woman said. The term stuck. From that moment on, Henry and Kate were our energy twins. They even looked alike, which, as they got older, pissed off both of them. They got tired of being asked if they were twins, and, after putting up with it for a while, they started telling people that they were indeed twins.

We completed our home in English Turn and moved there in 1995. Patti was five, Henry was two, and Kate was one. English Turn was a large, gated community built around a golf course. Kids roamed the streets like animals in a habitat, safe and happy. Henry took to it immediately. As he grew older, we were constantly finding him in the yard, exploring the boundaries of his new environment. Our house was at the end of a cul-de-sac, a foofy way of saying a dead-end street. It was a great place to teach Henry to ride a bike. At five, after seeing Patti learn to ride, Henry insisted he was ready. He would get on the bike and pedal while I held the handlebars and ran alongside yelling, "Keep pedaling. Don't stop." After a few falls and de minimis amounts of blood, he figured it out. Now, he was free to explore. He had a good friend, Forbes, who also lived in the neighborhood, so getting on his little bike, feet moving at a rapid pace, Henry would wobble down the street, unaware that we were following close behind. He was only five, after all. English Turn was safe, but you never know. By the time he was six, we were worn out from keeping tabs on him, so we set ground rules on where he could and could not go without us. I'm sure he pushed those limits, but what you don't know won't hurt you. I suspect we didn't know a lot.

Late on Sunday afternoons, when the golf course was empty, I would take Henry and Kate to ride with me while I played a few holes. They shared the passenger seat, fighting over who was taking up more room. When I got near the green, they would jump out and run through the sand traps, laughing as they chased each other. Luckily, no other golfers were around. The smiles and laughter of those Sunday afternoons have stayed with me. How carefree they were, untroubled by what would come. Happy to be with each other.

Since we had a big backyard, we got a full-size trampoline for the kids as a Christmas present. Henry was especially enamored with it. He would jump on it for hours, tucking his legs and then pushing down at the last minute to achieve maximum lift. All of the kids loved it, but no one more than Henry. I'm not sure why. Maybe it was the height he could achieve? The feeling of flight he felt? All I know was that the look in his eyes when he bounced really high was electric. It was mesmerizing. If he caught you watching, he would give you a sly smile. It was a smile with just a wee bit of devil in it. It was the smile that said I know something you don't know.

Henry was always an intense kid. Relentless, with a mind like a steel trap. Once you promised him something, the bars of the trap would come down, and that promise would stay there, trapped forever. He never forgot it. And he never let you forget it. You said it, you better make it happen. Even at a very early age this was true. With the two other kids, we could often put them off with a promise of "tomorrow." Not Henry. When he was four, he wanted to go to his friend Forbes' house to play. It was late, so I told him we would talk about it the next morning. I awoke the next morning to Henry's little face. "Dad. Dad. Wake up. Can we go to Forbes' house now?"

For vacations we would drive to our house in Santa Rosa Beach, Florida. Heidi and I had a video unit installed in the backseat so the kids could put on headphones and watch a movie. On one particular ride to the beach, we strapped the three kids into the back seat, and they watched *The Sound of Music,* one of their favorites. Each sported a set of headphones so that the three-hour movie translated into three hours of quiet time for Heidi and me up in the front seat. Driving along, thrilled with our decision to invest in what, at the time, was a state-of-the-art system, suddenly the quiet was broken. Henry, in a sweet little voice from the back seat was belting out the song that the nuns and the Mother Superior were singing about their wayward Maria. The lines from the song still ring in my ears:

How do you solve a problem like Maria?
How do you catch a cloud and pin it down?
How do you hold a moonbeam in your hand?

He sang completely happy, completely unaware of anything but the song. So engrossed in the notion of a moonbeam that he didn't notice we were all looking at him. It was both incredibly funny and endearing. Patti and Kate took off their headphones to listen and giggle at their brother. I'm sure he was just swept up by the beautiful song. And there's little doubt in my mind that as he sang those words, he really did want to know, how you catch a cloud? And pin it down? What is a moonbeam, and how do you hold it? Once he realized we were all looking at him, he gave us a sneer and quit singing out loud. But I could see in the rearview mirror that his lips were still moving to the words of the song.

Henry, like all our kids, went to preschool at Uptown Montessori, run by Martha Kabacoff. She had at least twenty years of experience running a Montessori program. She was well-versed in the art of dealing with kids and all their oddities. Henry's particular obsession was always having a clean shirt. Yet, given the way he would chow down food, this became problematic. Martha, in her wisdom, recognized Henry's quirk and suggested we keep a few extra shirts at school. Problem solved. There was, however, one problem she could not solve. Henry was a lover of maps. Heidi, encouraging this interest, had cut up a bunch of maps and used them as wallpaper for his bathroom. He loved that bathroom. He would sit in his bath, cheeks reddened by the warm water, staring at the walls. I guess he was imagining the world and how large it seemed. Always asking where this was or where that was. At school, a map of Africa hung where the kids kept their lockers. Henry wanted that map. He would ask a teacher every day if he could have that map. *Every* day. They kept saying we shall see, and every day he asked again. Finally, after six months of this, Martha was worn down and gave Henry the map. Relentless!

Henry was relentless, yes, but also an inquisitive soul. His favorite books were the DK books on birds and rocks and dinosaurs or any other earthbound thing. He especially loved dinosaurs and would quiz us on them constantly. "Hey Dad, what's the most ferocious dinosaur?" Before I could answer he'd say, "T. rex. I've told you that before." And he had, maybe once or three hundred times. One night I was reading to him a new book on dinosaurs. He was captivated by it, turning the pages faster than I could read them. He wanted to sleep with the book. Before handing him the book, I noticed on the back page it had been written by Kirk Johnson, Head of Paleontology at the Denver Museum and my college fraternity brother.

"Henry, I know the guy who wrote this book," pointing to his picture on the inside cover. "He's a friend."

"No, you don't," Henry said with a serious tone.

"I do. Next year when we go to Copper Mountain to ski, we can stop in Denver on the way home. I'm sure Kirk will show us the dinosaur exhibition."

Henry looked at me in awe, as if I was sixteen feet tall. It was as if I knew the Power Rangers, and they were on their way over.

"Yeah. I really want to go. Please call him," Henry said urgently. "Call him now."

The next day I called Kirk. It had been fifteen years, but it felt like yesterday. We reminisced about old times, the glory days of college. After about twenty minutes of recounting old stories, I told him about Henry and his love of anything pre-historic. I told him about our annual Mardi Gras ski trip and asked if we could stop by the museum the next time we were close to Denver. He said absolutely and that he was looking forward to seeing me again. Henry was thrilled.

The following year we took all the kids skiing. We dropped Patti off at ski school and put Henry and Kate in the Belly Button Bakery, which was nothing more than childcare on skis. Heidi and I went back to the condo and got ready to ski. The sun was bright, and the temperature was a balmy forty degrees. It had snowed the night before, and the mountain had a fresh sheen of powder like icing on a cake. We dressed and went out to take the lift up, Heidi by my side. I was looking forward to a great day. Our first run was like that first hit of coffee in the morning. It woke us up and got us ready for the day. On our next ride up, in the hut at the top of the lift, there was a sign that read: "Tripp and Heidi Friedler please call the operator." This was before cell phones and the only way to get a message to someone on the mountain. It was awful. Why would we need to call? What was going on? We skied down to a phone and called. The operator connected us to Belly Button Bakery. They told us that the energy twins had tried to escape but that Butch Cassidy and the Sundance Kid had been successfully detained. All the same, we had to go by and scoop them up. Heidi and I looked at each other in disbelief. There went our day. I was deflated as we went over to grab our little outlaws. When we got there, they had settled back down and looked up at us like the angels they were not. Big smiles escaped from the mound of clothes they were wrapped up in. Little bundles of love waiting for their heroes to return. We were not as happy, and they sensed that, making them smile even harder, as if their smiles alone could soften us. We gathered them up and took them back to the condo. Our ski day was over. The next day we convinced Belly Button Bakery to give them one more try. After a stern warning from us and a substantial bribe of hot chocolate, they agreed to go back. Leaving them did nothing to alleviate our concern. Every chair lift became tense as we neared the top, and then, not seeing our names on the board, we breathed a sigh of relief. No more escape attempts.

On the way to the airport in Denver, we stopped at the Denver Museum of Nature and Science. Henry jumped up and down, unable to contain his excitement. It was as if he was meeting Santa Claus himself. Kirk came out of his office and gave us a tour. He took us "backstage" and let Henry open various drawers and take out bones. Henry's exuberance was contagious, and everyone, even his sisters, enjoyed the tour. I can still see that smile. He was all teeth, his eyes as bright as stars. Pure joy. His dream had come true, and I was happy to be the guy who had delivered it.

While the kids loved English Turn, Heidi did not. She missed Uptown New Orleans and the convenience of proximity. In English Turn you're twenty minutes from anything, and twenty minutes from *everything*. All three kids were Uptown, at Newman School, and Heidi was growing tired of the carpools back and forth across the Mississippi River. Between her work and the kids, she was spending too much time in the car. It began to wear on her. I was not the most observant of husbands, but even I could see the toll this was taking on her. Unbeknownst to Heidi, I had started exploring houses back Uptown. After a few months of looking, I found the perfect house, three blocks from Newman. It had been on the market a long time because it needed a ton of work. But Heidi, with her amazing eye, could see the potential immediately. So, we put in a bid, and it was accepted. We were moving. The renovation would take a year, but we were excited to be moving back Uptown.

chapter 2

GREAT EXPECTATIONS

Outside Henry's childhood bedroom, greeting him day after day, was a picture frame holding two almost identical black and white photos. In a thin black frame with white matting, the two photos sat side by side like twin beds. In one, my great-grandfather, Joseph Friedler, and my grandfather, Frank Friedler, Sr., are standing behind an old wooden chair with a faded seat cushion. My father, Frank Friedler, Jr., is seated in that old wooden chair. He is holding me in his lap. I'm about two years old. Everyone is in a suit and tie. Well, everyone but me. I'm in some frilly linen jumpsuit that I pray I never wore again. My great-grandfather and my grandfather look deadly serious, not even a trace of a smile. They look as if they're standing at attention in an army barracks, ready for roll call. My dad, however, is smiling, and I appear to be happy too, notwithstanding the outfit. Next to this photo, separated by a one-inch strip of white matting, is a nearly identical picture with the same chair. Except in this one, I'm seated in the chair with Henry on my lap. He's no more than one, dressed in an equally frilly outfit we'd put him in for the occasion. My dad and my grandfather are behind us. It is a series of pictures meant to convey generational family history. It was the first thing Henry saw every morning when he left his bedroom. I wonder if some days it looked to him more like a cut that wouldn't stop bleeding.

Henry, always inquisitive, quickly became interested in our family history. Curious who the old men in the picture were, he would ask questions about them. Where did they come from? How did we end up in New Orleans? What was my grandfather like? Was he like his own "Pappy"? My grandfather died when Henry was six, and his memories of him were vague.

Growing up, my grandfather lived about a mile away from us on Audubon Boulevard. Frank Friedler, Sr., was a small man with a big personality. At family events, people would gravitate toward him. I would watch him hold court. People were taken by him, and I was too. Some of my earliest memories are going to visit him and my grandmother after Sunday school. And we had family dinners with them at their house every Thursday. He took time with me. He asked about school and my tennis. And he told stories. I was fascinated by the ones about his exploits on the lacrosse field. He had inherited the Family Bible, which had been handed down from his great-grandfather. He recorded every birth, marriage, and death in our extended family. I loved his stories about us. Sitting with him on Sunday afternoons with Henry by my side, I'd look over at Henry, wide-eyed and attentive. Seems as if Henry, too, was curious about our past.

Henry's full name is Henry Frank Friedler. He was named after the patriarch of our family, Henry Frank, my great-great-grandfather, who had come over to St. Louis from Eastern Europe in the 1850s. He'd moved around a bit in search of opportunities before joining the Union Army as a sutler. Sutlers were merchants who sold goods to the Union soldiers. He followed Grant's army down south and, at the end of the war, found himself in Natchez, Mississippi. There, he met a man named John Mayer. While John Mayer had no love of Yankees, he did have some Jewish daughters to marry off. John married his daughter Melanie off to Henry. Henry Frank settled in Natchez, started a family, and became a successful businessman. He and Melanie had twelve kids, but only three made it to adulthood, a boy and two girls. The oldest of his daughters was Ophelia Frank. By all accounts Ophelia was a force to be reckoned with. At around age eighteen, she was sent off to a conservatory in Boston, which was unusual for a woman in the late 1800s. When Henry Frank wanted to send his son, John, to prep school, he asked Ophelia to find the right school. It was Ophelia who started our centuries-old family tradition when she decided that her younger brother John should attend Phillips Exeter Academy. Upon her return home to Natchez from Boston, she met and soon married Joseph Friedler, from Vidalia, Louisiana, a tiny town across the Mississippi from Natchez. They had three boys of which my grandfather was the middle child. All three were shipped off to Exeter then Yale. All three settled in New Orleans after college. When Ophelia died in 1927, Joseph, now a widower, followed his boys to New Orleans.

Once, when Henry was thirteen, I took him to a tennis tournament in Jackson, Mississippi. But first, I had to make a quick stop in Baton Rouge for business. The easiest way to get from Baton Rouge to Jackson is through Natchez, so I asked Henry if he wanted to see where his ancestors were buried. Our whole Natchez branch is buried in the National Cemetery on a spot the locals called Jew Hill. It's on a bluff overlooking the Mississippi River surrounded by old oaks and magnolia trees. Prime real estate. We found the area, parked, and walked up the small hill. Beyond an ancient iron fence were about fifteen headstones spread around in a haphazard way. We found a break in the fence and went through. It was as if we had stepped back in time. There was nothing to discern the present, surrounded as we were by relatives from the past. We started reading the names on the headstones, saying them out loud. Ophelia Frank, Caroline Frank, Ernest Frank, Edgar Frank, Wilhelm Frank. Most of them died as children. Henry then wandered off on his own, looking at headstones and saying the names. A few feet from the old iron fence and in the center of the graves he found his namesake.

"Dad, I found Henry Frank," he called out excitedly, stopping at a large headstone in the center of all the others.

I walked over to him, and we stood together, taking in all the family history that lay before us. I took a picture of Henry next to Henry Frank's headstone with my iPhone. After snapping a few pictures, Henry grinned and asked, "What do you think Henry Frank would say if he knew we were taking a picture on a cell phone?" I just laughed.

What I knew, and Henry had yet to learn, was that our family had its secrets. And in our family, probably like many families, we swept those secrets under the rug, albeit a rug covered by more beautiful things. Our family's legacy, passed down through each generation, is that we are brutally demanding and deeply angst ridden. The best way to avoid any confrontation was to just succeed. Succeed in school. Succeed in sports. Succeed financially. It worked for me. Building upon my dad's success, I was able to achieve a level of success I never dreamed possible. My business had grown into something that provided my family with luxuries I never had growing up. My dad always said that all he could give me was "a name and an education, and what I did with both was up to me." I was able to do a lot. As it turned out, I was one of the lucky ones, though it did come with a cost. Heidi and the kids paid it, as I was always working. Striving to succeed. To prove myself worthy.

For the Friedlers, success was never measured in emotional terms but only by external metrics. I heard stories of my grandfather and his two brothers being summoned every January 1st, wives in tow, to their dad's house, where they were to report on how their year had been financially and what the next year's projections looked like. I often heard of the fear this inspired in my grandfather and his brothers. The annoyance of the wives, sitting there like schoolkids outside the principal's office. And I heard the stories of my grandfather as an all-American lacrosse player at Yale. His victories on the field, the articles in the local paper. I don't think I was told these stories by accident. It was impressed on me at an early age that if you were "successful," you might be left alone. Who cares if you're happy? The more important question: did you win? I was taught that winning was the goal at the exclusion of all else. Even happiness. We all got caught up in the hurricane of expectations, and Henry would have a tough time weathering that storm. Unwittingly, I made it tougher by blindly continuing our family tradition. But the fact that I was unaware of what I was doing was no excuse. Ignorance is not a defense.

It took me many years of living and countless hours of therapy to understand how difficult this force can be. How easy it was to get caught up in its seeming glory. When I was about twelve, we took a family trip to Boston. My father was driving, my mother was navigating from the front seat. Ancient times. No GPS or MapQuest. We got around using something called maps. As we tried to find our way to the Boston Aquarium through the winding streets of the city, we got lost. My mother, a huge map splayed on her lap, tried to get us back on the right track, but we just got more and more lost. And my dad got madder and madder. Finally, he turned to me and asked, "Tripp, do you know how to read a map?"

"Yeah, I think so." Even at that young age, I was cocky.

"Then get in the front seat and take over navigation from your mom. We're lost."

I was elated. My dad needed *my* help. I was being moved to the front seat. It was my moment to shine, and I loved it. Smiling so big it took up my whole face. I happily switched places with my mom. Only looking back now do I see that my moment of triumph came at the expense of my mom. How she must have suffered being made to feel less than. Her own son as eager co-conspirator. None of this crossed my mind. I was being called up to the big leagues and felt I was ready. From that moment on, I was the permanent navigator. I became the person everyone turned to for help, a role I have come to relish and dread all at the same time. A role that would have me navigating toward countless solutions for Henry down the road.

Henry was a smart kid if not yet wise, and the questionable lessons were not lost on him. It is the unspoken words that kids hear the loudest, the attention that gets paid when things are good, and the displeasure expressed at small failures. I expected good grades in school and success in athletics. Luckily, for him, Henry excelled at both. He could see the pride in my eyes when he won at soccer. I coached his team in the local ten and under soccer league. I was a demanding coach whose only goal was winning. I'm sure he could feel my competitive juices flowing right into his. We fed off each other in unhealthy ways, creating a dynamic that revolved around winning. The same as my father had with me. I was continuing a family tradition without even knowing what it was or why I was doing it.

School was no different. Like sports, school seemed to come easy to Henry. He never had to study much to do well, spending most of his time playing with his friends. Knowing that good grades would keep me at bay, he did just enough work to shut me up. We had an implicit, unspoken agreement: as long as he made good grades and won at sports, I would be happy. And so would he. In his early years, this was easy. As time went on, it got harder.

With his disease buried inside him, waiting to escape, I now wonder what effect all these expectations had on him. How much of his disease was nature and how much was nurture? And if nature, where did it come from? Some genes can be easily traced to specific diseases. Sickle cell anemia and hemophilia are two examples. Other diseases such as cancer, schizophrenia, or bipolar disorder are polygenic, being regulated by more than one gene and tougher to isolate. Thus, tracing the "nature" element of Henry's disease proved to be difficult. The Friedlers loved to talk about successes. But were there others among us whose history had been deleted like a bad fact? Relatives who didn't fit well into our carefully crafted narrative? No one really likes to talk about mental illness today. What must it have been like 150 years ago? Had there been clues? All I know is that the expectations Henry was born into, those two photos slicing into him each morning as he exited his bedroom, a place that would become his refuge years down the line, were something of a clue. Something powerful that I wish I had understood better back then.

chapter 3

PRACTICE?

We moved back to Uptown New Orleans in the summer of 2001. Patti was eleven, Henry was eight, and Kate had just turned seven. This house was our dream house, large, on a private street with only six other homes. A cul-de-sac hugging a neutral ground. The street only had one way in and out, the perfect place for the kids to play, safe from cars. The kids were happy that they each got their own bedroom and bathroom. Heidi allowed each kid to pick out the colors for their bedrooms, which pleased them. Although Heidi did retain veto powers. After all, she was a decorator. On the third floor there was a guest room, a playroom for the kids. an office for Heidi, and a small gym for me. The house had everything we wanted. Most importantly, we were only three blocks from their school, Newman. The commute would be easy, and the kids would get an extra forty-five minutes of sleep. Solid gold for them.

Sports have always played a central role in my life. For Henry it was the same. When we moved back Uptown, I joined the New Orleans Lawn and Tennis Club. I had played tennis for Amherst College and was excited to take it up again. Henry and Patti joined Carrolton's travel soccer teams, though Patti quickly tired of it. Henry, on the other hand, loved it. He was the center midfielder and one of the team's stars. His feet were quick, and, combined with his speed and aggressiveness, made him a baby-faced killer on the pitch. He loved traveling with his teammates, and soon, his favorite times were the weekends at hotels with his buddies. Henry hated losing but loved competition. And that boy would work the refs. He was always complaining that he was being fouled. There is a picture in my office taken by a professional photographer of Henry at one of his games. He is in his green-on-green uniform with his hair cropped short. A kid a head taller than Henry has the ball. Henry is looking to steal it and is behind him. His eyes are squinting, his mouth snarled. And while he was only eleven, he had the look of a raptor as it goes in for its prey. His right arm grabbing his opponent's arm, eyes on the ball. He had clearly been photographed in the middle of a foul. The proof was in the picture, like those dreaded red light cameras that catch you in the middle of the intersection, leaving no room for argument. Unless you are Henry. He and I looked at that picture one afternoon.

"That's not a foul," he said aggressively.

"What about the arm? Kinda looks like you are grabbing him," I said flatly.

"Nope. They never called a foul, so there was no foul. Don't know what you're looking at. That is a clean steal, Dad," he said in a firm tone indicating the conversation was over. He looked at me, then the picture, and knowing he was caught, laughed, and walked away.

Henry was the athlete I could never be. He could play any sport, but his favorite was soccer. He was fast, and his footwork next level. While, like me, he was a small child and a late bloomer (though he ultimately grew to be just under six feet), he was a gifted athlete with the rare combination of coordination, determination, and ferocity. A few years into my return to tennis, Henry wanted to take tennis lessons. I think he saw me enjoying a sport he imagined he could do as well. And maybe, like me with my dad, he wanted to do stuff I did. I'm not sure. But I was thrilled. I'd always enjoyed playing tennis with my dad, and now my son wanted to give it a go. A lifetime hitting partner! I can still vividly remember playing with my dad and how much joy that brought both of us. How proud he was of me and how proud I was that he was proud of me. How loved I felt in those moments. I was looking for the same with Henry. I was sure he would be exceptional. I dreamed of a Wimbledon in his future. I would live vicariously through his success. Be Top Dad to a Top Player. All these unhealthy thoughts coursed through me like a fever.

I found him a great teaching pro. As I'd expected, Henry was a natural. It was as if he had found a long-lost friend. He wanted to spend all his time getting better. He couldn't get enough, constantly begging me to take him to hit. The Friedler genes at work again. I would take him out to hit a basket of balls. While he wanted me to feed him balls, he didn't want any advice. He had always been headstrong, and tennis was no exception.

"Dad, just feed me balls. That's not what my coach says. What do you even know about tennis?" I guess the fact I had played in college was irrelevant. I was frustrated but understood. I was his dad, so what could I possibly know? I could have been Roger Federer, and it wouldn't have made a difference. I knew Henry was relentless, and I admired that in him. His stubbornness and his quest to be better fit right into our family dynamic. So, I let it slide. Henry worked hard at getting better and at least listened to his actual coach, if not to me. He made quick improvements and started playing tournaments right away.

In tennis, unlike soccer, you're out there by yourself, and when you lose there's no one else to blame. I could tell there was a joy in Henry on the soccer field that was missing on the tennis court. The pressure of being out there all alone would get to him. But he was winning more than he was losing and kept coming back for more. And he was good, moving around the court like a gazelle. I remember watching him play his first tournament. Another dad asked if Henry was my son. "Yep," I replied proudly, my chest out a little more than usual.

"Does he play soccer?" he asked. I was surprised he knew this. Now I was more curious than proud.

"Yes. How did you know?"

"Look at his footwork. You can tell," he replied.

His tennis, it seemed, benefited from his soccer, and he loved both. However, like a sixth-grade boy fawning over his seventeen-year-old babysitter, one of those loves remained unrequited. By age twelve his soccer coach was telling us that Henry had to commit to playing only soccer, or he would be cut from the team. The coach was concerned that Henry was missing practices, which wasn't fair to the other kids. He had a valid point. But it was only one practice a week. I couldn't understand the coach's hard stance. As Allen Iverson once said, "Practice? You talking about practice?" The coach was unmoved and unmovable. When I told Henry, he didn't understand.

"Why do they care if I do both? There's never a conflict between tennis and soccer matches. This sucks. Who's making me choose? You?" He was pissed.

"No. I think you should be able to do both. The soccer coach is the one who is making you choose. He says you're missing too many practices," I said, not even believing what I was saying.

"I've only missed a few, and I'm one of the better players. That's not fair. Plus, it is not like I'm goofing off when I miss practice. I'm playing tennis, which only helps my soccer. This is crap," he said as he walked away.

I agreed. He should have been allowed to do both. At least for a while longer. Why should any kid have to make such a choice at twelve? It was unfair, and Henry knew it. This was the first time Henry ran headfirst into an unforgiving system. Unfortunately, it would not be the last.

After thinking about it for a few days, he chose tennis, probably because he wanted to hang out on the courts with me. Even at the age of twelve, this was a critical juncture in his life. Henry loved his friends. And he had a lot of them. He was friends with the jocks. He was friends with the artsy kids. He was friends with the nerds. He was that kind of kid. That's why he loved soccer. It's a classic team sport fostering friendships and a sense of belonging. Tennis, on the other hand, is lonely. You're out there all by yourself. There's no one to blame and no one to help. The soccer coach could have allowed him to miss a practice once a week. If tennis were hurting his soccer, then bench him. And if Henry was riding the bench, then he could decide if his tennis was not worth it. It seemed unfair to make him choose. I know for certain he regretted his choice. Later in life he would bring this up to me. He told me that he wished he'd stuck with soccer. I didn't realize what the loss of a team sport would mean to him. I would have tried harder to convince the coach to let him stay and do both had I understood. I'm not sure why I didn't.

Henry quickly got over the anger at being forced to give up soccer and put his all into tennis. As he became even better, I grew more invested in his tennis. I would hit with him every time he asked. And that was all the time. I'd travel with him to every tournament, trying to pick him up when he lost and high fiving him when he won. Sometimes, it's tough with our children to separate us from them. Henry's agility on the tennis court made me proud. But there was more, of course. It gave me a chance to relive my tennis, albeit at a level I could never achieve. I knew Henry felt this pressure. There were the unspoken expectations of achievement that our family history demanded. And now this extra pressure that his dad, the college tennis player, was applying. Henry was hard enough on himself. This extra weight must have been like carrying around another twenty pounds. And he only weighed eighty.

Soon a darker dynamic emerged in our relationship, a dynamic rooted in his desire to seek validation from me. It would play itself out in the middle of matches. If he made a bad shot, he would immediately look at me and be angry if I showed even a hint of frustration. I became adept at keeping a poker face, or simply walking away when it became too much for me. While Henry won most, if not all, of his tie breakers, I didn't see a single one. Too much for me to handle.

While tennis is a solo sport, tournaments are a group activity. There was at least one big tournament a month in exotic destinations like Jackson, Mississippi, and Little Rock, Arkansas. There is nothing quite like Mobile, Alabama, in July. Henry *loved* going to these tournaments. There would be ten to fourteen kids who all practiced together. Given the outgoing kid Henry was, he soon became friends with most of the top players in Louisiana. He was extremely competitive, yet eager to form friendships with the other players. They would hang out, playing ping pong or cards or just watching each other's sets. After a match they would head back to the hotel and the swimming pool for endless games of Marco Polo. Then the kids, and a convoy of parents with their credit cards, would head out for dinner.

Watching Henry play was nerve-wracking, and Heidi didn't like it. That meant that I took Henry to most of his tournaments. We spent a lot of time together, and most of it was good. But it was never fun when Henry lost, which was most tournaments. In a tennis tournament, there's only one winner. Unless you're that kid, you end up learning to lose. Henry was not a good loser. He was gracious on the court, but once off it, it took him a long while to get over the loss. I understood this, of course. I hated losing more than I enjoyed winning, and Henry suffered from the same affliction, a victim of a family value system he could not see. I had never been taught to embrace failure as a natural part of life. Now, Henry was having to deal with failure, and he was suffering. He was a sweet boy with a fragility that was always there, lurking just beneath the surface. He hid it well, but at times I saw it. A false bravado masking a scared little boy afraid of letting people down. And it hurt me to see this. Instead of acknowledging it and talking about it, I did what I had been taught to do: ignore it, sweep it under a pretty rug. Instead of being cool with his vulnerability, I demanded more toughness. Instead of letting him know it was okay to fail, okay to be afraid, I pushed him to work harder, be better, to win. One time after a particularly hard loss, he shook hands then stormed off the court. He shot right by me and headed straight to the car. By the time I caught up with him, I could see his face was bright red. His eyes were little slits, his lips so tight I was surprised he could get any words out at all.

"I can't believe I lost to that kid. He sucked. I must have double faulted at least fifteen times. My serve is crap. Let's go. I need to go to the club when we get back and hit a bucket of serves." The tournament was in Baton Rouge about ninety minutes from home. I drove him straight to the club, so Henry could work on his serve. He was twelve.

chapter 4

SEA CHANGE

Henry loved music. We spent hours together listening to each other's favorite bands. Some of the bands I enjoy the most were ones Henry introduced me to: Cage the Elephant, Portugal the Man, and The Black Rebel Motorcycle Club. Even his old man slipped in a couple to his regular rotation. One of Henry's early favorites was one I turned him onto, The Red Hot Chili Peppers. I bought their 2006 album, *Stadium Arcadium*, when it came out, and Henry listened to it non-stop. "Dani California" was one of his favorite songs. When they came to town that October to play Voodoo Fest the year Henry turned fourteen, he *begged* me to take him. The night of the concert was a beautiful fall night in New Orleans with an almost-full moon. The place was packed, so he asked if I could put him on my shoulders for a few songs. Since he was still relatively small, I was happy to oblige. I looked up at him, his eyes wide at the whole scene. He kept asking me if that funny smell was pot. It was. I hoped it was a lucky guess on his part. But I suspected it was not.

Around this time, Henry started to become moody. He would still flash moments of the old Henry, listening to music with me, hitting tennis balls, playing scrabble with his mom, his funny wit on display. But I noticed his temper becoming short and fierce. And a kind of lack of joy. Heidi, of course, saw this too. Most times he was the kid we knew, but, more and more, Heidi and I began to witness a sea change in Henry. Where had my sweet child gone?

He seemed to be replaced by a new kid who never felt content. Heidi bore the brunt of his anger. She could do nothing right. If Heidi cleaned his room, he would yell that she needed to stay out of his room. If she didn't clean his room, he would yell at her for not doing so. He was like a schoolyard bully, and Heidi was the new kid in town. He would hang out at the computer, playing his music at thunderous levels, knowing it would upset us. I think that was his point. No slight was too small. I chalked it up to that well-established syndrome: Early Teenage Jackass. But there was more. As time went on, his whole personality changed. He wore a perpetual frown. He was angry all the time. Any little thing could set him off. If I noticed his shoes were untied, he would yell "So what? Leave me alone."

"But you might trip," I would say.

"Then I'll trip. How is that your problem?"

By the second semester of his freshman year at Newman in 2008, Henry was almost fifteen. He was no longer the fun-loving and kind kid we all knew. He hadn't yet hit puberty, but he was losing that angelic look. His baby fat gone, his face had thinned out, and his expression was almost always serious. His beautiful smile had disappeared, and an angry scowl had replaced it. His list of grievances kept growing. So much so that he even targeted his energy twin, Kate. He began to complain that it was unfair that Kate, who was dyslexic, got extra time to complete her tests. He argued that if he could have more time he would do better and that his grades, which had started to slide, would improve. He wanted whatever edge he could get. Like the kid in that soccer photograph, Henry knew he was pushing the edge of the envelope. He was so in the embrace of our family culture of winning at all costs that any means seemed to justify the ends.

As usual, Henry was relentless and worked hard in his pursuit of extra time on his tests. By the spring of ninth grade, Henry had worn us down, so we took him for a psycho educational evaluation—the necessary step to get extra time for exams. At Ochsner Hospital the psychologist did a complete analysis, putting Henry through numerous tests as well as interviewing us and his teachers. Reading that report today is haunting. The Friedler family's demand for top achievement jumps out at you like a ghost in a haunted house. It's hard for me to read and leaves me wondering why I didn't pay more attention to it at the time. It's like seeing a movie for the second time, annoyed that you didn't catch the plot twists the first time. The report makes clear the effect of being undersized had on Henry. I, too, had grown up smaller than the other kids. Middle school and much of high school was rough for me, but it just made me tougher and more resilient. Not so for Henry. The constant ridicule was getting to him.

His tennis career, while still going well, was also affected by his size, and what success he did have at tournaments around the South was not helping his status at Newman School. At free periods, he was no longer picked first or second for baseball, basketball, or football. Having not yet started puberty, he was self-conscious around girls who were already taller than he was. All of this made life a struggle, and, when he acted out because of it, I missed it. I'd invested in the hope that what Henry was going through was just classic teenager angst. But re-reading the doctor's report, it's clear that he saw a depressed kid who was struggling to navigate the perils of teenage life. The bullies and the girls, the cliques and the parties. The slights, real and imagined.

It's ironic that I was so willing to lie to myself about Henry and that Ochsner report. It was difficult for me to accept that my son was anything but perfect. Most times it is easier to lie to yourself than it is to accept a hard truth. In life, being clear-eyed about where you are is critical—though challenging. Most of us are well-versed in the art of self-delusion. It's like trying to make an airline reservation to New York without having the ability to tell them where you're leaving from. Can't be done. Until you know your own location, nothing is really possible. And here I was violating my own cardinal rule. I was in denial about my own son. It was a hard truth to face. So, I buried it. I told myself that Henry was just going through a phase. Hoping I was right. Worried I wasn't.

Heidi, more attuned to Henry and his strange vibrations,

was far better at sensing when things were wrong. Far better at all things emotional. I was a good salesman and getting Heidi to marry me had been my ultimate sale. We met at Tulane Law School in August of 1985. I was studying for the bar exam, and she was taking summer school classes. She was getting both a law degree and an MBA in a four-year program. We were in the student lounge of the law school when I first saw her. We made eye contact for about two seconds from across the room, but, in those two seconds, I knew that this was someone I needed to meet. I asked my friends if anyone knew her, and my buddy Sid said he did. He said that her name was Heidi Hackley and that he would get her number. Sid, a man of his word, did just that. Allegedly, the call went something like this:

"Heidi, a friend of mine wants to know if I can give him your number."

"Who is it? Do I know him?"

"Tripp Friedler. You saw him in the lounge. Short, Jewish-looking guy."

"Oh yea. I know who you're talking about. Sure. Tell him to call me."

I called and we went out. Our first date was sushi, which was a novelty in 1985, and then, we went to a small bar with music called Benny's, now long gone. The night was over far too quickly. I remember walking her to the door and giving her a three second kiss that sent chills down my spine. I can still remember, all these years later, exactly where we were and the electricity I felt. I left thinking maybe I should have tried to kiss her longer. It was all I could think about on my way home. I was hooked.

The next day I called again, and we ended up going out *every day* for the next six months. That's not an exaggeration. We spent every single day together. I was beyond smitten. But I had recently started practicing law and, as a result of my job, was miserable most of the time. And by most of the time, I mean all of the time. Heidi, tired of my grumpy complaining, had seen enough. She broke up with me in March, and we each went our separate ways on the dating carousel. That December, almost a year later, Heidi called. She was getting ready to graduate the following May and wanted to talk. She was having an existential problem about what to do with her life. She knew she didn't want to practice law but had no clue what to do instead. I like to tell Heidi that she just called me to get back together. And she likes to say, "That may be true, but you certainly came running." She was right. I did come running, and by January we were back together. And by September of 1987, we were married.

Heidi knew she didn't want to practice law, though she did take and pass the bar exam. Heidi had always been more of an artist than a businessperson, so it was no surprise that she found a job that catered to her sense of style. She started working with an interior designer right out of school. She knew she was talented, and everyone who worked with Heidi knew she was talented. And after Patti was born, Heidi decided it was time to start her own firm. She quickly grew it into a very successful practice. But her kids came first, and Heidi was an even better mom than she was a designer. She was the perfect complement to my overbearing nature, trying to soften me in ways that I desperately needed. Deeply intuitive and sensitive, she was usually right and would sense when things were wrong well before I had even the slightest clue.

Heidi was ready to accept that Henry was mildly depressed. She began reading everything she could on depression in adolescents and wanted me to do the same. She tried to get me to ease up on him and recognize his struggles. She felt I was too hard on him, that my constant pressing was hurting Henry. She wanted empathy from me, and all I came up with was more discipline. I thought I had it under control. Why would I need to read anything? I knew everything. And while I was no help, neither of us were aware of the storms brewing beneath the surface. The disease fighting its way out.

Henry was struggling to find his place in a world that continued to shift around him. His friends were all going through puberty, visibly becoming young men, and he was still a boy. His sisters continued to flourish. Watching his sisters thrive was hard on Henry. Patti was a straight A student, and Kate was one of the more popular kids, on her way to becoming head cheerleader. All of this was hard on Henry. He grew even more short-tempered and withdrawn. The Ochsner report clearly stated that he was being picked on for being short. Henry was a sensitive kid and the taunting got to him. Tormented him, really. At the time, I didn't see how bad it was.

Yet, Henry had something up his genetic sleeve. Little did his taunting friends know that his mother came from the Land of Giants! Heidi's 5'8." The smallest male on Heidi's side of the family was 6'. One nephew is 6'5." Luckily, Henry got some of those Hackley genes. Eventually, he shot up to be just shy of six feet tall. But he didn't have his growth spurt until he was seventeen.

We have a picture of him on the tennis team representing the Southern District for sectionals, where the top kids from one region play those from other regions. He was fourteen. He's the shortest kid on the team, including the girls. Looking back, it's enlightening to see how the same experiences shaped Henry and me so differently. Being small only stoked my fire and built up my resilience. But it all wore Henry down. At the time I was unaware of the pain he was carrying. Having gone through much of the same taunting, I thought I understood. But I only saw it from my own perspective. Instead of fully embracing that he was different from me, I failed to offer any help. I didn't see what was right in front of me. So, I never saw or anticipated what would soon push him into a crisis and pounce on him like a wolf on its prey.

chapter 5

PREP SCHOOLS

At the end of the summer of 2008, Henry was fifteen and entering tenth grade. Heidi and I had just dropped Patti off for her freshman year of college at Trinity College in Hartford, Connecticut. The school year at Newman was also just starting up, so Henry and Kate stayed home with our longtime babysitter Stacy. September is notoriously hurricane season in the Gulf of Mexico, and, as luck would have it, Hurricane Gustav had New Orleans in the crosshairs. After Katrina three years earlier, everyone suffered from a little PTSD. Seeing that menacing circular blob heading right for New Orleans, we decided to have Stacy put Henry and Kate on a plane to meet us in New York City. They caught the last flight out of New Orleans. We met them at LaGuardia and headed into Manhattan. Heidi and I had planned to spend a few days alone enjoying the city but were happy to have Kate and Henry join us. They were thrilled to have time off so quickly from school and happily shared a room in Midtown. We saw *Wicked* on Broadway and had some great meals. Henry and I got to see Rafa Nadal play at the U.S. Open. What a treat it was watching Henry watch Nadal, his mouth open and his head moving to and fro like a metronome as he followed the ball back and forth over the net. One time he caught me looking at him. Henry just smiled then went back to watching the match. It was such a nice break from the fighting and arguing and reminded me of what life had been like a mere year earlier. I didn't want the match to end.

We were stuck in New York for a few extra days, as the New Orleans airport remained closed after Gustav. During this down time, Henry confessed that he had been researching high schools and found a tennis academy in Austin, Texas, which was connected to a reputable school, St. Stephen's Episcopal. He wanted to go. He never told us why he wanted to leave Newman, though we had our suspicions from the Ochsner report about the taunting. I had visions of my son being a great college tennis player, so I didn't ask. Heidi, like me, had gone to prep school, so she was also open to his switching schools. Neither of us really questioned the urgency. At the time it seemed like the perfect solution. A fresh start for Henry. We contacted the school and arranged to fly straight from New York to Austin.

St. Stephen's is located on the west side of Austin. It occupies 370 acres of rolling land that opens onto Lake Austin. A spectacular looking spot, from a vegetation-rich canyon to bright green grasses along a pretty creek that runs through the campus, it looked more like a country club than school. The tennis facility was first class with twelve hard courts and two clay courts, as well as a state-of-the-art training room. Heidi and I both fell in love with the place and the people. We were sure this would be a good home for Henry for the next three years.

Henry visited with the tennis coach and the admission staff. He really liked the coach and everything he had to say. We could tell he was excited and really wanted to go. His eyes and the huge grin on his face said all we needed to hear.

"Dad, this place is great," he said, his eyes looking right into mine. "I really want to go here. They get people in all the best colleges. It's not just a tennis academy. Please let me go. Please!"

It was impressive. The scholastics were superb, and he would get top class coaching in tennis. The school informed us he could start immediately, with one caveat: Henry would have to repeat the ninth grade. Henry had an April birthday making him one of the youngest kids in his class. At the time we felt he was ready to start, even though there would be boys a full year older than Henry. With his late maturity and being younger than his peers, this gave us an excellent opportunity to reset. It was not something we could have done at Newman. Henry would never leave his friends to go back a year and be in his sister's class. Still, we were worried about how he would react to this, as he would graduate high school the same year as his little sister. But he was undeterred. Henry was so eager for a change in his environment that he agreed immediately. This quick agreement to stay back a year should have given us pause. It did not. We just wanted the joy back in Henry, so we were willing to believe a change of scenery would help.

The newness of everything was a jolt of electricity to Henry. His mood improved, and he was pleasant on the phone. We talked often, especially at the beginning. There were some very good players in the tennis program, and Henry enjoyed the competition. He became friendly with the tennis players and made some friends in the classroom as well. A few of Henry's better friends were part of the soccer program. That program was as equally well-staffed as the tennis program, and one of Henry's friends went on to be drafted into the MLS. Henry loved kicking the soccer ball around whenever he had a free moment.

But the freshness of the new school wore off quickly. After a few months, Henry began complaining about how his teachers were bad and that the weekends were boring. He was playing a lot of tennis, and it was wearing him down. About two months into his time at St. Stephen's and right before the Thanksgiving break, I got a call from Henry. He sounded down.

"Dad, this place is not like the day we visited," he quietly complained. "All the normal kids are day students. The boarders are the only ones left in the evenings. They hid all of them from us when we visited. I wish I had known that before I decided to come."

"Henry. They didn't hide kids," I replied. "You just came in the middle of a day and saw all the students, day students included. You told me you had friends. Go home with them on weekends. I'm sure they'd let you."

"They would, but I can't," he answered. "Tennis takes up most weekends. The tennis is nice, and I'm getting much better. I'm sure it will all work out. Dad, don't worry, I'm just venting. Tell mom hello."

That conversation stayed with me a while. While I was always trying to fix whatever problem anyone was having, I downplayed Henry's concerns, not even telling Heidi, keeping his complaints to myself. Once again, I stuck my head in the sand and convinced myself that everything would be fine.

Two weeks later he injured his wrist. Unable to play tennis, things went from bad to worse. While St. Stephen's was technically a boarding school, only about 10% of the student body were boarders. The rest were day students who left when classes ended. Now, with his tennis friends busy with tennis and his other friends off at their homes, Henry was lonely. And while the teasing and bullying had stopped, Henry missed his New Orleans friends.

By the end of the semester, Henry had decided he wanted to move on. He didn't want to come home, so he started looking at prep schools on the east coast. He realized he would need recommendations from teachers. Having only been there one semester, he had few relationships with his teachers. On top of that, because of the pressure he felt to make good grades, Henry had become a grade grubber. If he got a B, he would ask the teacher why and what he could do to get it to an A. He was relentless, and many teachers found this annoying. He had a tough time getting teachers to write recommendations for him. Some did, but they were less than enthusiastic.

His mood was worsening by the day. He would call most days with a new complaint: the food sucked, TV time was limited, his wrist hurt. The list went on and on. In retrospect, it was obvious he was suffering from a mild depression. He kept thinking that if he changed schools again, things would get better. Rather than deal with his problems, he was trying to outrun them. And Heidi and I were willing co-conspirators. We should have dealt with the real issue head on. Instead, we started looking for a new school.

As has often been said, you're only as happy as your most unhappy child. Henry was that child. His unhappiness was more than normal teenager angst. Both Patti and Kate had plenty of that. Henry's seemed deeper. Angst at his core. It concerned us. Depression is a tough illness to handle. This was my first brush with it, and I handled it poorly. I knew something was off, but, like Henry, I was all too willing to take the easy path. Neither Heidi nor I was willing to dig deep and figure out the true source of his unhappiness. Either unwilling or unable to tell Henry no, we set off to visit prep schools.

We visited many of the great ones, including Exeter. Henry would have been a fifth generation there, but Exeter rejected him. As did a couple of others that he visited. We started getting nervous. I had a close associate who suggested we look at The Lawrenceville School in Lawrenceville, New Jersey. We visited the school. We loved it. Henry got in. At Lawrenceville the kids all live in residential houses. My friend's had been Kennedy House, so we visited that one when we were there. Peter Becker was the teacher in charge of the Kennedy House. Henry and Peter really hit it off, and Henry asked if it would be possible to get in Kennedy when he started next fall. Peter told him that he would make that happen. Henry, once again, seemed excited about the future, making his last semester at St. Stephen's bearable.

The Lawrenceville School, outside of Princeton, has a 700-acre campus with rolling hills and spectacular views. The dining hall is large and elegant, and the kids all eat together as a house. In fact, the house system defined much of what you did socially at Lawrenceville. Henry joined Kennedy House. He loved it and quickly made good friends.

Each house fielded a football team to play tackle football in the fall. Kids playing for the Lawrenceville football team were not allowed in, so it wasn't as hard-hitting and violent as it might have been. The kids were smaller and a little slower. It was a good fit for Henry. Given his quick feet and aggressiveness, Henry excelled at this and was a starter on the team. Kennedy House even made it to the championship game. They lost, but the experience bonded Henry to his teammates in a way that fed his soul. He was still one of the smallest kids in the dorm, yet no one teased him. When we spoke on the phone, I could hear the smile in his voice. I traveled to New York often for business, and, since Lawrenceville is only an hour and twenty minutes away, I'd arrange my meetings in such a way that I could go visit Henry on the weekends. I could see he was happy. He seemed to know everyone. When we walked on campus, he would glide along showing me this place and that. As we walked around campus, he smiled in ways I had not seen in a while—those electric smiles I used to see when he was on the trampoline. His grades were also very good, and he was the second-best player on the varsity tennis team as a sophomore. He had a great tenth grade year, and, when he came home for the summer, he was the happiest we had seen him in a while. He would still get moody occasionally, but, overall, it was a good summer.

Henry, now sixteen and a rising junior at Lawrenceville, was excelling. My career was going well, and I was on my way to building a business I loved. I had written my first book about my approach to business called *Free Gulliver: Six Swift Lessons in Life Planning.* I had sold some copies and was genuinely content. As usual, right when things were at their best, everything turned.

chapter 6

STRIKE TWO, YOU'RE OUT

Each year there is a national conference put on by the NAIS (National Association of Independent Schools) for board chairs and their heads of school. They have speakers talking about issues related to private schools: fundraising, capital spending, school governance, and strengthening the overall board-head working relationship. In late October 2010, it was in Baltimore, and, being Board Chair of Newman School, I attended with Newman's Head of School, T.J. Locke. I was in a breakout session on capital campaigns when I got the call from Henry. I always take calls from my kids, so I got up and left the room in order to talk.

"Dad, I think I screwed up," he said in a crackly voice.

"What do you mean?" I asked, the concern obvious in my voice.

"A group of us were smoking some pot, and later that day someone told on us and all of us were forced to take a drug test. I knew I would get caught, so I tried to fake my test by getting a friend to pee for me. I got caught. They're saying they're going to throw me out."

He was crying. I could hear how broken he was, realizing the deep hole he had dug for himself.

"They are going to call you to come up here to get me if they kick me out. I screwed up bad this time. I can't believe I'm such a fuck-up. I love it here, Dad," he said frantically.

Henry was being so hard on himself that I felt no need to pile on. "Henry, try to calm down. I'm at a conference in Baltimore with heads of other schools. Let me talk to T.J. and see what we should do. I'll call back soon," I said as calmly as possible.

I was in shock. I knew I needed some help in navigating this from someone I trusted. It took me a minute to find T.J. He had become a good friend, and I knew I could count on him to help me figure things out. I found him in the lounge between sessions and explained Henry's predicament. T.J. was sympathetic. He knew the Head of Lawrenceville, who was also at the conference, and offered to talk to her. When he returned from his chat, I could tell by his frowning look that we had a problem. T.J. told me that the Head of Lawrenceville knew about the situation and had told him it was a real problem. Lawrenceville had a two-strike policy. The faculty wanted to consider this infraction two strikes, one for smoking pot and one for faking the test.

T.J and I both felt I should get up there as soon as possible. Henry would go before a review board consisting of both students and faculty. We were both hopeful that Henry would get a second chance, but I should be there for moral support. The rest of the morning was spent making reservations to get to Lawrenceville and talking with Heidi. While she desperately wanted to be there for Henry, she trusted me to get there quickly and do the best I could. I checked out of my hotel and took a short flight to Philadelphia where I rented a car for the forty-five-minute drive to Lawrenceville.

For the entire car ride up, I kept replaying my conversation with Henry. My nerves were shot when I got to Lawrenceville that night. I knew Henry would be a mess as well, and I was not looking forward to what was coming. When I got to Kennedy House, he was waiting on the porch. He ran up to me and hugged me. His eyes were red, and he kept saying," I really screwed up this time. I love it here. I can't believe I'm such a fuck up. God, what an idiot." It was painful watching Henry beat himself up. I tried to console him, but he was inconsolable.

The next day Henry and I walked over to the room where the review panel was assembled. I waited outside while he went into the room. Henry was sincerely contrite. More than anything, he wanted to remain at Lawrenceville with his friends. He'd worked all night on the speech that he had to give to the panel. I thought it was very good and felt sincere. Other than this incident, he had been a model student. He had good grades and played #2 for the Lawrenceville tennis team. He had never had any other discipline issues. Surely, they would give him another chance. The faculty was unmovable and unmoved. Henry was kicked out of Lawrenceville.

As his dad, this was hard for me to watch. From my vantage point, it seemed that Lawrenceville gave no weight to the effects this would have on Henry. They could have given him a second chance. They could have given him a less severe punishment and allowed him to grow from the experience. *That* would have been a real education, one that was in fact their responsibility as much as it was ours. School isn't just about getting good grades and getting into universities and on to good jobs. It's about learning to be part of a community that's larger than yourself. It's about embracing relationships that are easy and learning to understand the ones that are not. It's about questioning life's seeming certainties, including what's in the books and what the teachers teach, and then coming to your own conclusions. It is about preparing kids to enter the world as responsible, ethical, and moral human beings. Everyone is bound to fall short at some point in that process. Especially a sixteen-year-old. If you kicked out every kid who didn't get it right the first time without teaching him or her how to get it right, the world would be inhabited by billions of unevolved young men and women. How many kids have experimented with pot (and worse) and lied about it? And how about the teachers? I don't condone drug-taking in schools or lying about it. Not at all. But the punishment must fit the crime. First a warning, then a suspension, then expulsion. That seemed a reasonable course of action for what Henry had done. But Lawrenceville would have none of that. Two strikes in one pitch, and Henry was gone from the game. Hurt, embarrassed, and marked by the experience. It would have been traumatic for any child. For Henry, it was a disaster.

Henry crumpled with the news. Helping him pack his things hurt me to my core. He moved in slow motion as if unable to believe this was really happening. His friends would come visit one by one, just to be with him and try to comfort him. It was tough to watch. As each friend came by, Henry's shoulders dropped further, his despair on full display. Watching him say goodbye to his friends was like watching a funeral service. Sad eyes, head down. It was tough on both of us. Seeing my son so heartbroken tore me up. And there was little I could do to relieve his pain. He looked like someone who had just lost everything. His eyes moist as we drove away. I did my best to cheer him up, but the sense that he had failed us and himself would prove impossible that day. I knew this was a setback. And while it made Henry feel like a failure, to me he was still a successful kid. He was smart, a gifted athlete, and loved by his friends for his generosity and carefree nature. If the panel could have seen all the friends who came by to comfort Henry, they would have seen what I saw: a generous, kind soul who was still searching for his place in life. As much as I wanted to help, I felt powerless. It was like sitting in the stands watching your favorite team lose. Except this was my son.

We left Lawrenceville and went to a hotel. It was a long night, full of regret and angst. Henry's eyes were red from crying, and his shoulders sloped. He was already small, still only about 5'5", yet somehow, he looked even smaller. Our room had two queen beds, but Henry wanted to sleep with me. My usual instinct would have been to remain disciplined and say no, but I knew what he needed then was to be held and reassured, which is what I did. I wanted to let him know that I would protect him from the shitstorm that would be raining down on him. I knew his transition back to New Orleans would be rough. I did my best to comfort him, though I suspect I fell woefully short. He was returning home in circumstances none of us had anticipated. Newman School was willing to take him back, yet this was of little solace. Since he had stayed back a year when he went to St. Stephen's, he'd be returning to a class one year below his old friends. Worse, he'd be in the same class as his sister. While Henry and Kate were close, Kate would be the head cheerleader and get voted to the homecoming court. Henry was a kid who had just been kicked out of prep school.

That was a very quiet and depressing plane ride back to New Orleans. Henry wore a blank, faraway look. He was broken. I could clearly see it. And while his expulsion was an obvious setback, for some strange reason, I viewed it as merely an unfortunate event and not a failure of any kind. I still saw Henry as full of potential, brimming with talent and looks and smarts. Henry did not share my optimism. He was overcome with a sense of failure that I seemed unable to help him through. Could I have done better? Could I have prevented our family system from bearing down on him? Could I have done more to thwart the disease lurking inside Henry from escaping? My head says no, but my heart is not so sure.

I have always felt blame to be a useless emotion. Blame is the easy way out. It takes away all the hard work. Whether you blame yourself or others, all it does is absolve you from looking for the answers to the hard questions. Why did this happen? What could I have done differently? What is there to be learned? If you use blame to rationalize failures, then nothing can be learned. But blame is easier. It's the path most people choose. It was the path Henry chose.

chapter 7

BACK HOME

Upon his return to New Orleans, Henry was mad at the world. He was suffering the beginning of a severe depression and did not have the tools to ask for help. I didn't see the signs and was unable to offer any to him. Henry started blaming everything and everyone for his troubles. The first target of his wrath was Lawrenceville. Henry knew he had made a mistake. But he felt branded. Branded as someone not worthy of a second chance. And that devastated him. It was the beginning of a very long and dark road for Henry.

His return to New Orleans was hard for all of us. Teenage years are tough enough. Throw in a very public humiliation, and that takes it to another level. Henry was miserable, and he let everyone know it. Worst of all, he was mean to his energy twin Kate. He would pick on her and push her in ways he knew would hurt. He knew where her buttons were. He was mean to her friends when they came over to the house. He would make snide comments as to how she dressed. When she said something at dinner, he would tell her she was being stupid. Kate tried to brush it off, but we could tell it was getting to her. Kate fought back and their relationship deteriorated. The more failures he experienced, the meaner he got. And while his life was not going the way any of us planned, he did have some successes. He won the State Doubles Championship for Newman School and finished his junior year with decent grades. Yet, these accomplishments were overshadowed by his dark mood and his seeming indifference to everything.

I still felt that Henry had so much going for him. I could have done a better job of explaining that his one slip at Lawrenceville did not need to be a defining moment. I could have persuaded him to own it and create a new chapter, one that he would write instead of it being written for him. But I was unable to do so. I was unable to show him my vulnerabilities and my failures. No one had modeled this for me. No one had shown me how to help a kid navigate his way through and past his failures. I was as lost as he was.

Heidi and I tried to ease his return to Newman and raise his spirits. We were constantly trying to spin things in a positive light. Every day felt like a pep talk. He wanted none of it. Henry only looked for the negatives. His moods became darker and darker. Getting him to do any homework was impossible, and soon, we saw less and less of him. He would flee to his friends' houses where he wouldn't have to deal with us. His pot smoking got much worse. He seemed perpetually stoned.

Henry's life was admittedly tough, but Heidi and I paid a price as well. Being Chairman of the Board at Newman School, there were Newman parents and staff who thought that Henry was getting special treatment, and that Newman shouldn't have readmitted him. There were whispers at parties, looks at the grocery store. We felt we were being judged as lousy parents who were doing a poor job of raising our kids. This affected Heidi more than it did me. Heidi is loving and compassionate, a truly good person and a great parent. The sense of being criticized by our community had a toxic effect on her. She became depressed. Just going to the grocery store became a minefield. She worried that she was the subject of every conversation. And I couldn't convince her otherwise. I've always been a fixer, a solver of problems. Living with people who are sad or down is hard for me because my fixer mode gets activated, and I become relentless in pursuit of finding a solution. The problem was I, too, felt judged. People I barely knew would take it upon themselves to tell me what Henry "needed." One person I met at a business meeting told me all I needed was discipline and rules. He had three kids under eight and no experience with teenagers and their issues but felt perfectly confident in telling me how to handle my son who he had never met.

Most parents go through life doing the best they can. When you know someone whose child is having a rough time, you would like to think that could never happen to you. It's like pilots who are convinced that all crashes are pilot error, that had the pilot been more skilled, they could have prevented the crash. It's a survival mechanism allowing them to fly without fear. Parents use the same mechanism. You tell yourself that you are a good parent and that bad things don't happen to good parents. It was certainly the way I thought. As the great saying goes, shit happens. Circumstances just get the best of us, and then our humanity and our frailties are all too evident. I look back at it all now and regret that I wasn't able to communicate better with both Heidi and Henry. I was too busy hiding my own perceived failures—namely my inability to stop bad things from happening to Henry. I did not yet understand that much of this was beyond my control. So, I dug in and let the opportunity pass. Heidi got past the shame. Henry never did.

To make matters worse, there was Henry's inability to play any sports in his senior year. Since he had repeated ninth grade at St. Stephen's, he was technically in his fifth year of high school at Newman. In Louisiana sports, high schoolers are only allowed four years of eligibility. I could understand that Henry could not play another year of tennis. He didn't want to play any more tennis. He wanted to play soccer, a sport he had never played in high school. He had no years of prior soccer and just wanted the camaraderie of being part of the team. I could finally see why soccer had been so important to him, and why he had been so angry when forced to choose between tennis and soccer. It was clear now that he had chosen tennis to please me. I had been too happy with his decision to see that it came at a great cost to Henry.

We wanted to help him fulfill his desire to play soccer. Heidi and I were hoping one small win could get him back on track. I contacted Newman to see what we could do to get him eligible. It required a waiver from the Louisiana Athletic Association (LHSAA). The Athletic Director at Newman was supportive and applied for the waiver. He said it was a long shot but was willing to try. A hearing date was set. Henry, the athletic director, Heidi, and I all went up to Baton Rouge for the meeting. Watching Henry in that meeting was heartbreaking. He sat there as the Athletic Director made his case, hoping against hope that the system would not fail him yet again. His eyes glued on the panel, head tilted as if silently pleading for things to go his way. Unfortunately, the bureaucrats at the LHSAA had no empathy. They didn't even ask one question, their minds already made up. They held fast to the lazy "rules are rules" decree. Rules are rules only if the powers that be decide to enforce them without compassion or nuance. As a parent I was hoping they could see Henry and realize what a difference it would make to him to be able to join the team. As a parent you don't want to create a kid who is entitled. You want them to learn that rules matter and need to be followed. Yet, this rule seemed arbitrary in this case. Sometimes small things matter. Why can't adults in charge of kids take some time to discuss the nuance of a case? Had they done so, they could have seen that Henry was not violating the spirit of the rule. They could have seen what a crushing blow it was to Henry. Instead, they took the easy way out. I don't know if they harbored any ill will. All I know is that they didn't ask any questions. They didn't seem to want to know anything about him. And without comment, they crushed his dreams.

The ride home was quiet. None of us spoke. Henry put on his headphones, and I watched him suffer another defeat. I could tell he was upset that the adults in control of his future could be so unconcerned. I felt powerless. The one thing I wanted to give my son was a shot at redemption, and I couldn't even do that. A small gift to give to a kid who had been so beaten down. What harm would it have been to allow him to play one year of soccer? It wasn't like he was a star player who had been recruited. He was a lonely kid looking for a chance to be part of a community where he felt seen and wanted. He was looking for a road back. Why are we so hard on kids who have stumbled? What about our society makes us so inflexible? Why is it that our educational system doesn't seem to want to take any time to consider the needs of the very kids who need help the most? Sometimes it's just the smallest gestures that make a huge difference in someone's life. These were just a few of my thoughts during our silent drive home. I'm pretty sure Henry was thinking the same thing.

The rejection made the remainder of the school year tough. Henry drifted further and further away, like a boat in rough seas that has lost its anchor. He would come home from friends' houses with red eyes and a tired look, no doubt from hours spent smoking pot, and head straight for his room. His grades were plummeting. It was as if he had quit on life.

All this was taking its toll on my relationship with Heidi. Heidi is a "highly sensitive person" (HSP), a term first coined by psychologists Elaine and Arthur Aron in 1996 in their book, *The Highly Sensitive Person.* A highly sensitive person is thought to have an increased central nervous system sensitivity to physical, emotional, or social stimuli. It is said to affect about 20% of the population. I am not part of that 20%. This caused us to treat Henry in very different ways. Heidi could feel his pain in ways I could not. When I chose tough discipline, she would opt for compassion and forgiveness. She felt that my harshness was damaging Henry and pushing him farther and farther away. I saw her coddling of Henry as a direct assault on my authority. I felt she was undermining me. Refusing to see her side, I fought against her constantly—and I seldom fought fair. Fighting to win at all costs is not a good way to save a marriage. Especially when you're on the wrong side of the issue. I believe deep down I knew that my approach wasn't working. Again, in hindsight, I should have seen the signs. His mood was growing darker, which I chalked up to his anger at the system. He fought with me frequently, and I handled it poorly. Any little thing provoked a fight.

Passing Henry in the hallways as he was headed out to see friends, I'd say something insignificant: "Henry, that shirt has a hole in it."

"So what," he would reply, instantly on edge.

"Don't you think you have better choices?"

"What are you? The fashion police?" he snorted. "I can wear whatever I want to wear."

I felt disrespected. I would get mad. He would get madder. It was like a nuclear arms race, each party trying to outdo the other with bigger and more toxic missiles. There seemed to be no end to it. Heidi pleaded with me to be gentler with Henry. While he also picked fights with her, she could let it go. Not me. She felt that I was a big part of the problem. She was right, but since I'm always right, I didn't see it at the time. I personified the adage "you can be right, or you can be happy." I was convinced that Henry was just slacking off and that what he needed was toughness. This put a tremendous strain on our marriage. Every time I tried to discipline Henry, he and I ended up yelling at each other, which led to Heidi yelling at me. Feeling attacked, I dug in deeper. I was veering out of control, wrecking everything around me but too proud to admit I might be wrong. It created terrible tension, and all of us were unhappy.

Years earlier I had started seeing a therapist, Andre S., on some issues dealing with my dad and his Alzheimer's diagnosis. He had helped me work through those issues, so I continued to see him weekly. I began to discuss Henry with Andre. As much as it pained me, I knew Heidi was right, yet I continued to fight. Andre tried to help me work through my stubbornness. But it was hard. I had never been shown how to express vulnerabilities. Resilience was the only thing that counted in my family. I'd mastered that and expected Henry to follow suit. Only he wouldn't and couldn't, and I felt helpless. I hate feeling helpless. So, the cycle continued. Heidi tried her best to help me, yet I saw this as an unwanted interference. She asked me repeatedly to talk to Andre about Henry. And after every session, she would grill me on what he had said.

Finally, and in frustration, I asked her to come and ask Andre for herself. This turned out to be a great idea. Andre saved our marriage. Even today, Heidi calls our time with him "happy hour." He helped us to see each other's point of view. We were able to work through most of our issues with Andre as our mediator. I learned how to fight fair, a crucial tool, as Henry was becoming harder to handle. We began to see that we were on the same team and though we had different strengths and weaknesses, working together was the best route to take. The only route to take.

Henry was now a senior. He had given up on his grades. His only interests seemed to be smoking pot and pissing us off. He got straight A's at both. He spent more and more time in his room listening to music. Through all of this, he continued playing tennis, but his intensity was not there. His body was on the court, but his mind was elsewhere. Even with little effort, he did well at tournaments, excelling on sheer talent.

Getting thrown out of school is not so great for college applications. Neither was attending three high schools in five years. Henry's grades had tanked, his attitude sucked, but his saving grace was his tennis. He was recruited by at least one Division 1 school and many Division 3 schools. We visited some of these schools, and Henry decided on Colorado College in Colorado Springs, a great college that is very difficult to get into. The tennis coach told him he would get in he if applied for early action, and he would be a starter on the Varsity team in his freshman year. The snowy mountains around Colorado Springs were a bonus as Henry loved to ski. He was excited and applied immediately.

We were on our Christmas vacation and had missed our connection home. It was one in the morning, and we were exhausted and frustrated with our layover. While we were checking into our hotel, Henry opened his email to look for an update on the status of his Colorado College application. And there it was. I could see the excitement in Henry's eyes. Finally, some good news. Heidi and I watched as he clicked on the email and saw his smile disappear. He was rejected. We were incredulous. How could this happen after what the coach had said? What could have gone wrong? His grades, while not great, were okay, and his SAT scores fine. Henry had been assured by the coach that his tennis would overcome any shortfalls. This news rocked Henry. It felt to him that his future was irreversibly screwed by his one mistake at Lawrenceville. It was too early in the morning to call his college counselor. We tried to get some sleep, but Henry was dejected. It was an excruciating night. When we finally returned home, we spoke to his college guidance counselor. He spoke to the Director of Admissions at Colorado College, who said he would look into it and get back to him. A day later, the Director of Admissions called and told the counselor that they'd accept Henry if he committed right then. But Henry felt slighted and, in his fragile state, was no longer interested. I tried to convince him that it had all been a big mistake and that he should go, but he was firm. This excellent college was no longer a part of the plan.

chapter 8

COLLEGE LIFE

Henry squeaked out of Newman and into the University of Oregon. The summer before college in New Orleans was slow and hot. All summers in New Orleans are. And ours was full of constant bickering. Kate had been admitted to a great design program at Miami University of Ohio. She would start her freshman year in mid-August, and we could tell she was eager to escape and leave the turmoil behind. The fighting and constant tension had worn us all down. Dropping her off at school was a mix of emotions. We were sad to see our youngest flee the coop and happy that she was finally free from the chaos. Her broad grin and relaxed state let us know that she would be fine. Watching her interact with her new roommate and her new environment gave us the strength we needed to return home.

The closer we got to bringing Henry to Oregon, the happier he seemed to get. With only Henry home now, the tension eased a bit. Heidi and I planned a trip along the Oregon coast after we dropped Henry off at college. I wanted us to get our mojo back. It was a much-needed respite, one we were looking forward to. Finally, we would be empty nesters, and we were hopeful that we could get back to some sort of normalcy.

We dropped Henry off in Eugene on a Thursday. He had made it clear to us that he wanted a single. The University of Oregon put most freshmen in doubles or triples, and we'd had to get a psychiatrist to write a note to the school saying Henry needed to have his own room. I had a single my freshman year and thought nothing of this request. Blinded once again by my own history, I didn't see it as out of the ordinary. And in our desire to provide him with his own version of happiness, we created an environment that wasn't good for him. The only dorm with singles for freshmen was on the outskirts of campus about a half-mile away from the other freshmen dorms.

Henry was thrilled to finally start college. Heidi did her magic with the drab, sterile room and, after a few hours of rearranging and decorating, it looked bright and full of life. She had me running to and fro to get things done. She wore both me and our credit card out. Henry's excitement radiated from his face and lit up the whole room. He was getting a new start and was eager to make the most of it. Dropping our girls off at college had been a mixed bag, our anxiety in leaving them alone running headlong into seeing their excitement about their new worlds. Henry was no different. He was smiling ear to ear, ready to start a new life with new friends. He nudged us gently out of his room.

Heidi and I drove down to Gold Beach on the coast in southern Oregon. We planned to stay at the Tu Tu' Tun Lodge for two nights, then drive along the coast to Cannon Beach, and fly home from Portland. Heidi and I had not had any time to ourselves, and we needed to reconnect. The lodge was in the middle of nowhere, exactly where we wanted to be. We slept with windows open to the sound of crickets chirping and awoke to birds singing. We slowly remembered what we liked about each other. Between Heidi's smile and the beauty of our surroundings, I settled into a relaxing few days.

All that changed when I got a call early Sunday morning. It was Henry's cell phone. Seeing his picture popping up on my screen made my stomach turn. No college freshman ever called their dad at 8 a.m. on a Sunday morning just to chat.

"Henry, what's up? A little early to be calling your dad," I said jokingly.

"You're not going to believe what happened, Dad," Henry said, his voice both groggy and incredulous.

Not a great opening line.

"Dad, did you know that it's illegal to have an open can of beer on the street? "When did that law change? We do it all the time in New Orleans."

Henry had been arrested the night before for drinking a beer out on the street before the Oregon football game. Growing up in New Orleans, it is a staple of our lives to be able to carry an open drink on the streets. He'd used his fake ID (also a staple of New Orleans high schoolers) to buy beer for his new friends. He opened one on his way out of the store when he was stopped by the police. The officer had told him he couldn't do that, and Henry had said it was cool, he was twenty-one and happy to show the officer his ID. Poor Henry had no idea that didn't matter. As Cream once sang, "if it wasn't for bad luck, I would have no luck at all." That was Henry. He had spent all night in jail, and, to make matters worse, he had had a marijuana pipe on him. They'd given him a ticket for that as well. He ended up spending the next two weekends in two mandated courses for his offenses, one for alcohol and one for drugs. No frat parties, no football games, no hanging out with new friends. Instead, Henry spent his first two weekends in college learning of the dangers of drugs and alcohol. His college career was off to a booming start. And things went downhill from there.

Oregon, known for its grey skies and long winters, is an incubator for depression. With his dorm isolated and his tennis career over, Henry became depressed. It reached the point that he finally went to see a doctor on campus. That doctor prescribed the powerful anti-anxiety drug Klonopin.

At the same time and unbeknownst to us, Henry had started playing poker. What began as a way to make friends and kill time turned into something more sinister. Instead of going to frat parties, he soon discovered, unfortunately, his knack for poker. He spent more time playing poker than he did studying. And while his poker winnings went up, his grades went in the other direction. His depression deepened. I suspect he stopped taking his medication, and the only time he sounded half decent was when he won at poker. His moods became tied to the game. After a big win he was happy. After a bad loss he was low for days. When the school year ended, it was clear to everyone that Henry needed to come home. He applied to Tulane and was accepted. We were grateful for yet another chance, and hopeful that things would get better. Again, we would be wrong.

Henry started the new semester at Tulane in a dorm about a mile from home. He had a pleasant roommate, and Henry seemed content. He made new friends quickly and settled into his new college life. However, he was smoking a lot of pot, which his roommate disliked. Marijuana was my drug of choice in college, so I never worried too much about his habit. I thought it much safer than alcohol, I still do, and I didn't feel the need to monitor Henry's use of it. Once again, I was viewing the situation through my own history. I should have been firmer on him. I wasn't. The end result was that his roommate wanted Henry to move out. Henry took this as well as could be expected and ended up in a single in the same dorm. Problem solved. Or so we thought, until we got a call from his advisor saying Henry wasn't going to class. If he didn't improve, he would be asked to leave Tulane.

Henry was assigned a counselor to help him overcome any challenges. Jennifer was in her early thirties, not yet a decade removed from her own college experiences. She met with Henry twice a week, to talk about the stresses of college. She asked him what was going on in his life. But Henry was reluctant to talk about his issues. She called us to see if we had any insights. She clearly cared about her students and Henry in particular. We met with her in her small, cramped office on campus to see how we could help. We were deeply concerned, of course. For the first time in a while, we felt that we had a team in place that could help Henry. She was willing to do whatever it would take to get Henry back on track. The three of us met with Henry together. He assured us he would change. Agreeing to be supervised by his new counselor, Henry was allowed to come back for next semester. And then the shit hit the fan.

chapter 9

IAN

Henry had continued to spiral. There's nothing like getting a phone call from your twenty-year-old son as he stands twenty stories above the muddy Mississippi telling you he had almost jumped. And now, lying in bed with him as he fell asleep, my brain was in overdrive. I kept thinking about Heidi, waiting alone in our bedroom for me to emerge, drowning in thoughts of what could have been. Anxious for me to try to explain what went wrong. I was lost. I opened our bedroom door and heard her crying. Henry's near miss had awakened another wound. She could not bear to lose her second son.

Ian Armstrong Friedler was born on February 13, 1989. He was our first child. It had been a hard birth, and Ian developed a staph infection immediately after. He was confined to the Neonatal Intensive Care Unit of Baptist Hospital in New Orleans for the first two weeks of his life. Walking out of the hospital to go home without our baby was unnatural. Everything about it felt wrong. Heidi was constantly going back and forth to see Ian in the hospital, each time returning without her baby, her eyes red and moist. I tried my best to keep everything together.

Our neonatologist was Juan Gershanik, a no-nonsense doctor whose competency and confidence instilled in us a sense of guarded optimism. He called twice a day and brought us up to speed with Ian's progress.

Dr. Gershanik usually spoke to both of us. One day he spoke to me alone. "Triiiiiipp," he said in his Argentinian accent, "The next twelve hours will be critical for Ian. He will either be going home in a few days, or he might not make it. I didn't want to worry Heidi, but I need you to know."

I was in shock. Had I heard him right? How could this be happening? This was a very heavy load to carry alone, and I needed to share it with Heidi. I just had to find a way to tell her without scaring her any more than she already was. In the backyard, later that day, Heidi seemed as relaxed as I had seen her since Ian's birth. I felt it was as good a time as any to tell her the news.

"Heidi, there is something I need to tell you," I said, scared to keep going, "Dr. Gershanik told me the next twelve hours will be critical for Ian."

"What do you mean critical?" Heidi asked, her voice at least three pitches higher. "What exactly did he say?"

"He said that Ian was close to fighting off the infection and that within twelve hours he'll be fine, or his condition will worsen. He was optimistic but frank. It was scary," I said, doing my best to remember exactly what he had said.

Heidi's eyes filled with tears. "How can that be? I thought he was doing better. None of this makes sense." Her voice rising and cracking at the same time I stepped toward her. I needed to wrap her up and give her the confidence she needed. I held her tightly and whispered in her ear, "It'll be alright. I just know it." She wasn't buying it. We called Dr. Gershanik so she could ask him all the questions I was unable to answer. It was four hours after we had talked, and he had better news. Ian would be fine and should be able to go home with us in another five or six days. It was as though Heidi grew three inches and someone had given her a happy pill. The weight had been lifted and she was back to her old self. We immediately went to the hospital, so we could both hold our beautiful baby boy.

Those next six days flew by as we made plans to bring Ian home. We called Heidi's parents to let them know. They were eager to come down from Chicago to see their first grandchild. My dad and stepmom were equally thrilled to see their first grandchild, as only parents had been allowed to visit Ian in the hospital. Ian came home on February 19, 1989. My dad and Pam came over, and we passed Ian around like he was a precious family heirloom. Everyone wore huge grins. Ian gooed and gawed for the crowd. Heidi's parents arrived the next day. No one could stop holding him. For the first two weeks he was home, he was always in someone's arms. Our world was whole. Our family had started.

Ian was the joy of our lives. At the risk of sounding cavalier about my profound love for Heidi, I don't think I had ever loved anything as much as I loved my son. I know Heidi felt the same way. While I loved Heidi, I was enthralled by Ian. And I was the father. Heidi's bond must have been even stronger.

We would take Ian for strolls in the park after I got home from work. Weekends revolved around Ian. In our friend group, Ian was the first to be born, so weekends were full of visitors and more strolls around the park. Each day Ian got bigger and stronger. He would lie in his crib and raise his head, a feat we found Olympic athlete amazing. We had gone from the lows of Ian's hospital stay to the heights of joy at his every little move and sound and look. I remember going for a walk with Ian and Heidi down Henry Clay Avenue, near Audubon Park. It was early May, and the weather was beautiful. The sun had set around seven, and, after an early dinner, we took Ian for a stroll before bedtime. I joked with Heidi, "I could lose you, but, if anything ever happened to Ian, I would be devastated." I'm sure she felt the same. She was just too nice to say anything. Three weeks later our world imploded.

We were visiting my grandmother, Ethel Toor, in Palm Beach Florida for Memorial Day weekend. This was her first and only great-grandchild, and she had desperately wanted to meet Ian, paying for our trip and even buying a crib for the guestroom. We arrived on a Thursday afternoon, in time for an early dinner. After dinner she held Ian until it was time for him to be fed and put down for the night. Heidi nursed him and put him to sleep around eight. After putting him down, Heidi joined me as we visited with my grandmother. Around ten o'clock, we all went to bed.

The scream that woke me up the next morning was deafening. Thirty-four years later it still blasts through my memory if I allow it to, transporting me back to that room. I shot up in bed and saw Heidi leaning over the crib. Ian was blue and not breathing. He was cold. He was dead. Just writing about it all these years later turns me cold and numb. My world fell out from under me. It was hard to remain standing. I stopped breathing and everything went silent. I lost my bearings as my life as I knew it crumbled. I felt myself sinking, unable to save myself from drowning. It is a feeling permanently burned into my brain. One I will never forget.

The next few days involved a bunch of logistics. How to get Ian's body home? Where would the service be? What clothes would he wear in the coffin? It still remains a blur. Among the many horrible things associated with Ian's death was the inability of anyone to tell us why he died. The official cause was SIDS (Sudden Infant Death Syndrome). A SIDS diagnosis means the doctors had no idea why he died. As science gets better, the number of SIDS cases has declined. Maybe in today's world they could have given us a cause. But in 1989 it was SIDS. This only deepened our pain. We were left alone to imagine the many ways this might have been our fault. The guilt crept in, battering our already fragile states. Heidi was inconsolable. It took us many years and lots of counseling, but we were able to get through the tragedy with our marriage intact.

The years went by, and our family grew. We had never told our kids about Ian. They were still young, and we were concerned about their understanding of death. Navigating life as a child is hard enough, and we didn't want to make it harder by introducing death into the mix. We waited until they were ten, seven, and six to tell them. The truth was we were worried they would hear it from someone else.

We decided to take them to lunch, tell them about Ian, and then go to the cemetery to show them Ian's grave. We rehearsed many times what we would say and how we would say it. We gathered them all in the den one Friday afternoon when I got home from work and told them the plan.

"We're all going to lunch tomorrow at that restaurant Uptown by Gram and Pappy's on Magazine Street. The one by the fire station," I said.

They were immediately suspicious. We never went to lunch as a family.

"Why are we doing that?" Patti asked, leaning in for the answer.

"I wanted to ride bikes with Forbes tomorrow," Henry said.

"It'll be fun. Consider it an adventure. Mom and I want to talk to y'all, and we figured we would make a day of it. Henry, you and Forbes can ride bikes later, after we get back."

They bobbed their little heads in agreement, but we could tell they weren't buying it. Especially Patti, who was old enough to know something was up.

The next day we left English Turn and headed into the city. They peppered us with questions the whole ride there. We parked the car, and everyone piled out, eager to sit down and eat. We found a long table in the back and sat down with Heidi and Patti on one side and Henry, me, and Kate on the other side. One of us always had to separate the energy twins! What started as play between those two would often devolve into fighting and now was not the time. We ordered our lunch. The moment we finished ordering, Patti piped up, throwing me for a loop.

"So, what is it you want to tell us? Are you two getting divorced?" Divorced? Were we fighting so much that the kids thought divorce was even possible? Although the stress of three kids, a big house, our jobs, and a long commute was not a recipe for uninterrupted bliss, we were a far cry from divorce.

"No. Mom and I are not getting divorced," I said. "We love each other and love y'all. We would never do that."

Patti was confused now. What could this be all about? Then she started to smile as if a lightbulb had gone off in her head.

"Are we going to Disney World? That would be so much fun," she said, beaming.

Henry and Kate heard this and got very excited. "Yeah. Disney World! That would be awesome," they said in unison.

"No, we're not going to Disney World," I said.

"Why not?" Kate asked. This family gathering was getting away from us quickly.

"Mom and I wanted to tell you something, and we're sure you'll have lots of questions. Before any of you were born, we had a son named Ian who died when he was three months old."

Getting that out took every ounce of strength I had. No one spoke for what seemed like minutes but was probably fifteen seconds. There was complete silence. I sat and waited, as if I'd thrown a pitch and was waiting for the batter to line one back at my face. I was getting ready to say something else to break the awkward silence when Patti spoke.

"You mean I'm not the oldest?" she said incredulously.

"You're telling me I had a brother?" Henry asked with a sweet sincerity.

Heidi and I had to laugh. All that anxiety about telling them, and they just made it about themselves. Kids do say the strangest things. And often the wisest.

We finished lunch in an upbeat mood. The kids were excited when we let them order ice cream for dessert. The day was looking up. We paid up and set out on our way to Lake Lawn Cemetery, about fifteen minutes away. As we drove, the kids turned back to their questions, this time all about Ian. What did he look like? What happened to him? Where is the cemetery? What is a cemetery? On and on it went. Heidi and I were amused and already exhausted. More importantly, we were relieved. This had gone far better than we thought.

We arrived at Lake Lawn Cemetery and drove to our family plot. We have a single, large tombstone with the names of all of those buried there engraved on that tombstone. Patti was named after my mom who died of breast cancer when I was twenty-three. She is buried there, and Patti was excited to see her name in print, even if it was on a tombstone. Then, they saw Ian's name, but by this time they were over being at a cemetery and ready to be home. On the way home it was quiet in the car. I would like to think that the kids were contemplating the day. At the very least I was sure they were fascinated that the world was not as they had thought it to be. It turned out to be a positive experience for all of us. It taught our children that they could trust us. And they learned that they had a big brother, Ian.

chapter 10

GETTING HELP

And now, twenty-five years later, we'd come close to losing another child. The idea was unbearable. I walked into our bedroom, where Heidi stood in front of our bed, her eyes red, mascara staining her face. She asked a thousand questions, rapid fire.

"How was he? What did he say? What do we do? How close did he come?" and then she broke down crying. She had already lost one son. The thought that she had come this close to losing another was too much. *Actually*, unbearable. I walked over to her. We held each other and cried.

After a minute we let each other go, heads down, deep in worry. Henry had a problem. We had a problem. Yet, we had no answers, and no idea how to find them. Heidi kept asking what we should do, and I kept shaking my head in disbelief. This was well beyond my level of expertise. I told her that I thought we needed professional help and that tomorrow we would call Andre first then my friend John Denegre. John and I grew up together in New Orleans. He was a successful child psychiatrist who lived and worked in Montana. Between the two of them, Heidi and I were hopeful we could come up with a plan.

The next morning, I woke up early. I peered into Henry's room and saw he was still sleeping. Anyone who has watched a child sleep, whether they are three or twenty-three, knows how serene they look. There's a love that sweeps over you that is powerful. I wanted to crawl back into bed with Henry and hug him some more, but I knew he needed to sleep. I went downstairs to make coffee. Waiting for the coffee to brew, I sat in the kitchen staring at the walls, wondering what was next. Against the sound of each drop filling the coffee pot, my mind raced with jumbled thoughts, replaying the previous night over and over again.

Thirty minutes later Heidi came down. We sat together in shock, neither of us speaking. Finally, I broke the silence and suggested we should call our therapist Andre at nine. John was in Montana and an hour behind us, so I suggested we wait a while longer to call him. We desperately needed their advice.

We could hear Henry stirring in his room. In a few minutes, he came down into the kitchen. He had changed clothes and looked calm, even nonchalant. He didn't say a word as he went to get something from the refrigerator.

"Henry, we're going to have to talk about last night. Your mom and I are worried," I said.

"What are you talking about?" Henry said with acid-like disdain. A good night's sleep had allowed him to regain his defiance and contempt. "You're both such drama queens. You're blowing this way out of proportion."

I lost it. I'd had enough. "What the fuck are you talking

about?" I shouted at him. "You call me from the Mississippi River Bridge crying, telling me you almost jumped. Are you going to try to act like that never happened? We need to get you some help. I'm going to get us an appointment some-where, and you're *going* to go. Case closed. End of discussion." He stared at Heidi and me for a second, sneered then went back up to his room. I heard the door slam. A well-placed door slam was Henry's way of saying fuck you.

I called Andre at nine and left a message. I called John at ten and put him on speakerphone, so Heidi could hear as well. I told him what had happened and asked him what we should do. John had trained at the famed Menninger Clinic when it had been in Topeka, Kansas. The Menninger Clinic was founded in the 1920s by Dr. Charles Menninger and his sons, Doctors Karl and William Menninger. It was consid-ered one of the premier places for those suffering from mental health issues. In 2002, Menninger announced its affiliation with Baylor University, and in 2003 it moved from Topeka to Houston. John felt that was the best place for us to go. After I told him about our conversation with Henry, he agreed that we handled it correctly and that Henry needed professional help. Andre called back an hour later. He'd seen mixed results from Menninger's but also felt that was as good a place as any to start. Both agreed we should get an appointment with The Menninger Clinic in Houston as soon as we could.

We did a little research ourselves and were impressed with everything we read about Menninger. The clinic agreed to see Henry the following week. Henry didn't want to go but knew we wouldn't take no for an answer. We left for Houston a few days later.

The Menninger Clinic occupies about fifty acres of prime Houston real estate. The reception area was a new building with tall ceilings and huge windows. The place was awash with light, instilling a feeling of both light and lightness. The setting alone lifted our spirits and inspired confidence. We checked in, and the receptionist gave us a schedule that spelled out what the next three days would look like. The only thing on the agenda for Heidi and me was a one-hour meeting with a therapist after lunch. We hung out and read while a therapist took Henry for testing. After a lunch at a nearby Mexican restaurant, Henry went for more testing, as Heidi and I were ushered into a therapist's office. Our session with the therapist should have been a clue as to what was to come later. Heidi and I had very different takes on what was going on with Henry. We argued a little, occasionally correcting each other. And we would interrupt each other. But while Heidi and I approach things differently and are both strong-willed (one of us more stubborn than the other), we have a love and respect for each other that has withstood a lot of hard times. Including, of course, the death of Ian.

The therapist at Menninger didn't see that. The therapist insinuated that our marriage was in trouble and that the stress of our bad marriage could be impacting Henry. We didn't have a perfect marriage. Who does? But Heidi and I had worked hard on our marriage long before our issues with Henry.

I still remember the evening in the fall of 1997 when I came home from work and Heidi informed me that we needed to go to group marriage therapy. I was shocked. We had a perfect marriage—or at least I thought so. Clearly, when the kids had thought our "Ian lunch" was about divorce, they had intuited something that I had been too thick to sense. Heidi wasn't happy. I know I worked hard and sometimes left little room for Heidi and the kids. While I might not be the most empathetic person, I am devoted to Heidi and to our family, so I went to marriage counseling. Through that process I learned that I could be difficult to live with. I wanted to make Heidi happy and improve our marriage. We learned that often what we say is not always what our partner hears. We learned that tone is crucial. We learned to better communicate our feelings and to listen with open ears. When this Menninger therapist questioned our marriage, both of us were dubious. But we didn't say anything. This was about Henry, and we wanted to have an open mind to all the possibilities. Neither Heidi nor I believed our marriage was the problem

For the next two days, Henry went back for more tests and interviews. On the final day, the therapists would meet with us after lunch to discuss their findings and their suggestions. The lead therapist came to get us from the waiting room and led us into the same small room where he had conducted our interview the first day. He kept looking at a stack of papers in front of him. Then he told us that Henry's main issue was his use of marijuana. They suggested he enroll in their rehab program. I was shocked.

"What about his suicide attempt?" I asked incredulously. "Where does that fit in? Are you telling us that the root cause of all his problems is his marijuana use? How does that explain his recent trip to the top of the Mississippi River Bridge? What about his obvious depression?"

"We see kids like Henry every day," he replied in a condescending way. "Kids will use drugs to help navigate life. We believe that if he were to get his drug use under control everything else would improve."

I didn't buy it. Neither did Heidi. No mention of his obvious depression. I knew he smoked a lot of pot and we weren't happy about it. But I had also smoked a lot of pot. I had friends who had smoked a lot of pot. And I don't think any of us had contemplated suicide. Heidi and I had a kid who had just tried to *kill himself*. Pot seemed the least of our problems. What I wanted to say was, "Are you shitting me? We just spent three days running test after test and this is your call? Cool it on the pot?" But instead, I said nothing—very uncharacteristic for me. Heidi was also bewildered by this assessment, but she, too, remained quiet.

The therapist could see that we were trying to absorb what he had said. He could see that we weren't about to put Henry in rehab at that moment. He suggested we go home and think about it. We left the facility. We were drained. We felt abandoned by the professionals we desperately needed. I called

John, who had recommended Menninger's, and he was upset as well. In looking back, I don't think Henry's marijuana use was helpful to him. I also believe it was nowhere near the root cause of his issues. We were desperately looking for answers and had brought Henry to, allegedly, one of the best psychiatric clinics in the world. And all they had for us was that Henry was addicted to pot. We were deflated.

We returned to New Orleans with more questions than answers. Henry withdrew from Tulane, and we began looking for alternatives. We decided to try Outward Bound, a program designed to educate and build confidence through challenging outdoor activities. Their mission is to change lives through problem-solving and discovery. A course from September to November offered canoeing and backpacking in the Yucatan peninsula in Mexico. We all felt this would be great for Henry. Including Henry.

It was a quiet two months in New Orleans. With Henry safe in Mexico in the capable hands of Outward Bound, Heidi and I were able to take a beat. He had a great experience, returning to us exhausted and excited at the same time. He was ready to give Tulane another go, and we were eager for him to try. Like the parents of addicts, parents of kids suffering from mental illness are looking for any answers that might come their way. We were more than willing to believe that he was better, and all would be good again. We just wanted Henry to have the college experience we both had. We were sad that, thus far, he hadn't had it. After his Outward Bound program (which gave him a few college credits), we were looking for something to keep him occupied until Tulane started in January. We just wanted him safe and happy. He had expressed interest in yoga, so we sent him to a short yoga retreat near Carmel, California. He came home tanned and relaxed. He was sociable with his friends and nice to Heidi and me. It seemed like 2015 would be a good year after all. Then the wheels came off, again.

chapter 11

MESCALINE

Henry was twenty-one but still in his sophomore year of college at Tulane. He was living at home, and he seemed out of touch with the Tulane social life. He started hanging out with his New Orleans buddies from Newman, who had already graduated from college and were looking for work. Henry wasn't happy to be living at home, making little or no effort to spend any time with me or Heidi. He was moody and difficult to be around. We kept our distance and hoped things would improve.

It was a beautiful Sunday morning in February of 2015, sunny and not too cold. I was leaving to play tennis, and Heidi was already out running errands. As I left the house, I saw John and Steve, two of Henry's good friends from Newman, emerging from John's car. Henry was on the front porch waiting for them. They waved at me in passing. They were all laughing, but I couldn't hear what they were talking about. Believe me, I tried. They went inside, and I drove off.

I got back a couple of hours later, and John's car was still there. Heidi was home by now. She told me that Henry and his friends had been on the third floor all day just hanging out. We were pleased that he was hanging out with friends, and Heidi and I each went about our day. Later that afternoon I was watching college basketball in our family room when I heard Henry escorting them back downstairs and out the door. He'd been outside with them for about fifteen minutes when Henry came back in. He plopped down on a couch near me. He was wild-eyed, his hair everywhere. He wore a strange grin.

"Dad, what a great day," he said, almost shouting. "We all took some mescaline, and I'm still tripping!"

What?! Henry and I had the kind of relationship where he could share most things with me. I believe Henry knew deep down that I wouldn't judge him, and, as a result, he seemed very comfortable dropping this bomb on me. I was not. I had always had an internal debate about how much of my earlier life I should share with my kids. They all knew I smoked pot, but I kept my other drug experiences to myself. I felt certain that was not the sort of thing one discusses with one's kids.

"You took what?" I asked. "Why would you do that? Where did you get it from? Whose idea was this?"

Henry seemed agitated by my questions. "What's the big deal?" he said dismissively. "Mescaline is natural, anyway. The Indians use it to get in touch with their true self."

"Their true self?" I asked incredulously. "Where did you get the drugs? Where do you even get mescaline?"

"We ordered it off the internet," he answered.

"The internet! Are you crazy? How do you even know what you are getting? When did you take them?"

I was both furious and amazed at his naïveté.

"Dad, why are you being like that? It's a natural way to

get in touch with your true self. I'm seeing things in ways I've never seen before. Why are you being such an asshole? I'm out of here!" he said, and then he stormed out of the house, slamming the door behind him.

He was gone before I could even process what he had just said and done. Moving from pot to mescaline is a big jump. Hallucinogens are serious drugs, like going from a bicycle to a motorcycle. The stakes are a lot higher.

After I regained some composure, I tried to call him, but there was no answer. After an hour or so and Henry still not home, I told Heidi what had happened. She was not happy, to say the least. Having lost one child, she had always been overly protective of her children. "We have to go find him," she said. "What happens if he's in trouble? Call him now and see where he is. Can't we track him on his phone? Did you try that?"

"I've already tried calling," I said. "No answer. And for some reason the tracking is not working. Maybe he ran out of juice."

"We need to get in the car now and start driving around," Heidi said, close to a total panic attack. "Start calling his friends. We need to find him."

I was also beginning to panic, but knew her plan was not going to work. New Orleans is a small city, but it covers a lot of ground. He could have been anywhere. Driving around looking for a tripping kid on some street corner didn't seem like a good use of our time. He'd come home eventually, I reasoned, and we absolutely needed to be here when he did. We would just have to wait him out.

Heidi, knowing I was right, was upset. "Well, what are we supposed to do then? *Nothing*?" She was clearly mad and much of her anger was directed at me, as if this was all my fault. I tried to calm her down, but she was in no mood. "I'm going upstairs. *Do something. This is our son.*" Then she stormed out crying. A few seconds later I heard our bedroom door slam shut. That seemed to be an important form of communication in our house. I was left alone in the family room wondering what I had done wrong and how I could fix it. The TV was still on from earlier, as I sank into the couch and stared blankly at the images.

A few hours later, Henry came home looking even more disheveled. It was early evening by now. His hair was even wilder, and his clothes looked like they were about to fall off him. "Where have you been?" I asked as soon as he walked in the family room. Heidi, having heard the front door open and close, came down the stairs and into the room. Still distraught, she demanded to know where he had been. Henry just teed off on both of us.

"Just leave me alone. You both are incredible. You just can't stand to let me be me. You have to control everything. I'm going upstairs to bed," he said angrily, then bounded upstairs into his room and slammed his door shut. Another fuck you.

Heidi and I were left alone in the den just staring at each other. She was furious with me.

"I can't believe you knew about this and didn't tell me right away," she said icily and stormed out.

I was left alone with my own anxieties. Maybe he did have a drug issue. Maybe Menninger had been right all along. Maybe I should have taken a tougher stance with his pot smoking. Maybe I should have done more. Maybe, maybe, maybe... These thoughts and others raced through my mind, weighing on me further.

I went upstairs, where Heidi was already in bed and made it crystal clear to me that the conversation was over. I was hopeful that the next morning, I could talk some sense into Henry and calm things down. I had a tough time sleeping that night. I took a Klonopin and eventually fell asleep.

I woke up early and went downstairs to get some coffee. As soon I came into the kitchen, Henry appeared, startling me. It was clear from his appearance that Henry hadn't slept. He was in the same clothes from the previous day. He seemed off in a way that I'd never seen before. Like his mind and his body were in two different time zones.

I tried to start a conversation. "Henry, did you sleep last night?" I asked gently, trying not to upset him.

"Nope. Too much stuff going on that I need to fix to get any sleep," he said in an amped up voice. "Sleep is overrated anyway, I'm not even tired, did you know that mescaline is what Indians use to communicate with their past, I spent last night tapping into our family history and it's *fucked up*, no wonder you're so uptight." There was no punctuation between these sentences. Everything came out rapid fire.

It was 7 a.m., and I was in no mood for a lecture from my

son. Yet, even in my annoyed state, I could see that something wasn't right. I tried to calm him down, but the calmer my voice got the more frantic he became.

As he headed for the door he said, "I'm going to see Andre and tell him how he can fix you. You need help." And he was gone.

I was confused. What had just happened? There was no way he was still on mescaline. While never having done mescaline, I was pretty sure that a trip didn't last almost a full day.

A couple of hours later, Andre called me. He said that when he had arrived at the office Henry was waiting on his porch and wanted to talk about me. It seemed he had walked the two miles to Andre's office. Andre said Henry was extremely agitated and wasn't making a lot of sense. I told him about the mescaline. Andre agreed that the hallucinogen had probably run its course. That the mescaline alone couldn't explain Henry's state. Andre was deeply concerned and that worried me even more. This was a new situation for me. He was acting in ways I had never seen before.

I hung up with Andre and immediately called Henry's friend John, whom I knew better than Steve. John told me that they had indeed ordered the mescaline online and that he and Steve had had a normal psychedelic experience and had come down from their high. John was concerned about Henry. When they had left him, they were still a little high, but everything seemed fine. Hearing my description of Henry worried him.

Henry stayed in this altered state for a few days. It seemed he had slipped from a mescaline high to a more permanent altered state. I was confused. What could this be? I later learned that this was his first manic episode. It is unnerving to watch someone in the full throes of a manic episode. Henry's hair was an oily, tangled mess as he had not showered or slept in forty-eight hours. He wore the same clothes for days, and his eyes were the size of saucers. His voice was high-pitched. Watching him it seemed like he was experiencing everything for the first time. He looked like a child in a constant state of amazement. He would finish a sentence with a sentence with another sentence, like his brain was sprinting but his mouth was jogging. And what was coming out made no sense. His ideas were hard to follow at a normal pace. At a full sprint, impossible. I had never seen anything like it. It's like watching your favorite movie, but the characters are speaking Japanese and moving backward. You are seeing it and hearing it and utterly unable to process what is going on, though you feel certain that you *should* know because it i*s* your favorite movie. Throw in that this is happening to your son, and your own lostness is multiplied. Nothing made sense to me, yet everything seemed to make sense to Henry. He thought he had unlocked the answers to the universe, ready for whatever came his way. The person talking to me looked like Henry, but it wasn't Henry. It was *beyond* unnerving. Watching your son fully awake and spouting nonsensical garbage is a waking nightmare.

I turned to his mescaline co-conspirators for insight. Steve wasn't as helpful as John. He was downright hostile. He was irritated that I had convinced John to give me the rest of the drugs. He accused me of being a typical adult who didn't understand his own son. He went so far as to write me a letter telling me how little I knew my son and how I should just "chill." Steve told Henry he should "watch out for me."

Later that day, Henry asked John for the rest of the mescaline.

"I gave it to your dad," John said. "He was upset and worried, so I caved and gave it to him. Sorry."

Now Henry was both manic and furious. A very bad combination. Not only was I having to fight my son, but I was also having to do so with his accomplice, Steve. It was not a fair fight. "Give me my mescaline," he yelled after confronting me. "That's mine. John had no business giving it to you. I'm going to call the police and say you stole it."

Call the police? If he hadn't been so erratic and so angry, I would have laughed. "Yep, go ahead and call the police and tell them that your dad has your drugs and won't give them back. Curious how that will go over."

He was manic, not stupid. As this was his first manic episode, I had no idea what was going on. I later learned that bipolar disorder is a mood disorder defined as a person suffering from both depression and having had at least one manic episode. It is biological in nature and takes over the brain. Clearly Henry, who suffered from depression, was having a manic episode. His brain was in overdrive, and his thoughts were bouncing around like a pinball machine.

It took two more days for Henry to finally sleep. Sleep is the great elixir, the only thing other than medication, that will help bring a manic episode to its conclusion. I used to believe that mania was like a drug for the manic person. That they wanted to avoid sleep like the plague. That's far from the truth. The manic person doesn't see the need for sleep. Their brain won't *allow* them to stop. Like the police at the airport gesturing at you when you try to park, the brain wants you to keep moving. The brain becomes a force greater than you, telling you that sleep is the enemy. Thus, the mania continues. The thoughts keep racing. And while a manic episode was a nightmare for those around Henry, it seemed like nirvana for him. It appeared to us that he was experiencing a sense of euphoria. He thought he was the smartest person in the world. And everything was crystal clear. Sleep was an enemy to Henry. He fought that enemy for three days until he could fight no more.

The truth was that neurologically he couldn't sleep. Mania is a neurological bonfire, and, until it goes out, sleep is not an option. This is just one of the insidious natures of the disease. When he finally slept, he slept for twelve hours. He woke up better. Once again, he seemed fine. And once again, I lied to myself. I hoped that his reaction to mescaline was just a bad trip. He wasn't sick so much as he had simply taken a bad batch of drugs, I told myself, conveniently ignoring the fact that his friends had not reacted in the same way. Why let facts get in the way of the story I needed to believe? I didn't have a mentally ill child. That wasn't possible. That only happened to other people. I could fix this by keeping any form of hallucinogenic drugs away from him.

I was in deep denial.

chapter 12

ESCAPE FROM THE JUNGLE

We withdrew Henry from Tulane once again. As it turned out, for the last time. While there were no more manic episodes, his depression had gotten even worse. We took a ski trip to Copper Mountain during Mardi Gras. We said Henry could bring a friend, and he did. Henry, who loves to ski, spent most days in bed, leaving his friend to ski with me. We ignored the sleeping elephant in the room and tried to have a good time, but it was obvious that Henry was in trouble. When we returned home, his depression morphed into anger. He didn't want to live at home anymore. He was tired of me monitoring his sleep, checking on him every night and every morning. While I knew by the light on in his room that he wasn't sleeping well, I nevertheless repeatedly asked him how he slept. Even though I didn't yet believe he had bipolar disorder, it was clear that something was definitely off. The lack of sleep was making him more off.

My constant monitoring angered Henry. We fought all the time. All the fighting and Henry's troubled state put a major strain on all of us. We all tiptoed around Henry, trying to avoid the daily fight he was looking to pick. Attempting to stand my ground and fix this, I drew lines in the sand: when he needed to go to sleep, to wake up, to exercise, to job hunt. Henry crossed these lines every time. Each time felt like a direct assault on my authority. I felt that I was being attacked existentially. That by challenging my authority, Henry was questioning my whole being. I yearned for the respect I had had for my father and the respect he had had for his. But Henry wouldn't give it to me. And I blew up. Not a very mature position to take. Like a four-year-old yelling for cookies he couldn't have, I acted like a child. And, since the child in me needed so much to be admired, he came out with such force that I forgot I was the adult, the father, and Henry the sick child. Was Henry really testing me, or was that in my mind as well? Henry might just be being Henry. Maybe this was all my issue, not his.

Unafraid, he went toe to toe like a heavyweight boxer. On top of all that Heidi seemed to always take his side, which further annoyed me. I had to fight two people trying to push past emotional barriers that I refused to address. I was in way over my head. So, when Henry told us he wanted to get his own place, I jumped at the chance. It was time to take care of myself, and I needed the space to figure things out. I wanted to be part of the solution instead of part of the problem. Heidi was more circumspect. She was reluctant to let him loose in the world. But I convinced her to give it a shot, and, against her better judgement, she agreed. I'm not sure I convinced her as much as I wore her down. I was like a bulldozer clearing everything out of my path. If I bore down hard enough, I could will Henry to be well. Stay off the drugs and get back to normal. Or so I thought.

We found Henry a studio apartment Uptown near my office, on the ground floor of a building on Magazine Street. While the neighborhood was nice, the building was not. He had a first-floor apartment facing the street. It was about 600 square feet with no attractive qualities whatsoever. There were only two windows, one with real glass, and the other made from glass block, the kind you can't see through, the kind that lets in very little light. Heidi did her best to brighten it up, but there was very little that could be done. But Henry didn't care. He was happy to be on his own. We felt bad for him. He should have been in college, at a frat party having fun. Instead, he was in a dingy apartment with no light, to go along with his dimming prospects. As happy as we were to get our lives back, we also felt guilty. Had we rushed this for our own sanity? We pushed those feelings down, trying to remember that Henry wanted to live on his own and was unconcerned with appearances. Nonetheless, it was disheartening for Heidi and me.

When he moved to his new place he started working. He taught some tennis and delivered some food. We paid his rent and his utilities so all he had to cover was food and incidentals. He never asked for money, so we assumed he made enough. There were no more manic incidents. He would come over from time to time to eat a free meal with us. We would take him to some of his favorite restaurants to stay in touch. We hoped that things were moving in the right direction.

But living alone with no structure wasn't good for Henry. We monitored his phone and could see his locations. I watched the blinking blue dot move up and down Magazine Street. We were never certain if the movements were part of the normal course of his day or manic roaming. I became obsessed with Henry and his movements. All day, every day, I was worried about where he was or what he was doing. I couldn't escape his gravitational pull whether he was living at home or on his own. In a constant state of anxiety, I would find excuses to walk by his place, hoping to catch a glimpse of him. I never saw him.

After about two months of this, Heidi and I decided to go by his place and check on how he was living. Unbeknownst to Henry we had a key. We could tell by his phone that he was out, so we became two spies on a mission. He was about ten blocks away, so we knew we were on a tight timeframe. We went in. The chaos of his place was shocking. Trash everywhere. The bed unmade with sheets hardly covering the mattress. Pots on the stove, caked with god knows what. The roaches seemed to be the only ones enjoying the conditions. We looked at each other in disbelief. Living here was unthinkable for us. Yet, this was where Henry spent his time. Though we tried, we could not unsee the squalor.

We were frantic. We went home to discuss what we should do next. We knew we couldn't tell Henry we had been there. This was a violation of trust that would not be forgiven. We did what we always did when we had no answers. We called Andre, and he agreed to see us the next day.

Factoring in that we needed to find a place Henry would be willing to go, Heidi and I immediately began searching for programs that specialized in mental health. This greatly limited our choices. We knew Henry loved the outdoors and especially anything close to water. We finally found a place that we thought might satisfy our needs and be a place Henry would accept. Pure Life in Costa Rica specialized in young adults and adolescents using outdoor adventure therapy as a treatment tool. They considered it a course of study, one semester long, over three months. Like Outward Bound, they offered college credit. Their team used outdoor and adventure activities to help with depression, anxiety, and substance abuse issues. Their belief was that activities such as surfing and rafting help students develop confidence, self-esteem, and life skills to cope with the ups and downs of day-to-day life. Henry loved to both surf and raft, so we were hopeful he would agree to go. We printed out the material from their website and went to meet with Andre. He agreed that it sounded like a good place, and, after talking with them, he was even more convinced. Our next step was to convince Henry.

"Henry, if we could find a place you'd like, would you consider going on another trip like Outward Bound?"

Henry was dubious. "What do you mean? Like what kind of program? Why do you and mom keep harping on these things?" he asked with trepidation. "I'm fine. I can play poker and deliver food. I can take care of myself. Plus, I know I have other money from some sort of trust fund, but you're such a control freak you won't give me any. If I go to a program, will you let me have some of *my* money?"

Henry did have some money in a trust. He had once seen a statement addressed to him at our house from the trust company. He had opened it and seen how much he had. Unfortunately for him, he would not get the money until I died.

"Henry, I've told you repeatedly that the money in your trust is only yours when I die. And no, you cannot have access. But we'll pay for you to do this course in Costa Rica. It's a semester long and you'll get some college credit. Plus, they have surfing there."

Henry's curiosity was piqued. He had started surfing in Oregon and loved it. Also, we had been on vacation in Costa Rica years before, and Henry had loved the rain forest. He agreed to go. It was expensive, $20,000, but, fortunately, Heidi and I had the money. We felt it was money well spent if it could help Henry and give us a needed break. The semester started in two weeks, which was just in time to get tickets and passports handled. We coughed up the money and off he went.

When he left, we had to clean out his apartment—the first of four apartments we would have to pack up for him. It was heartbreaking each time, to be so up close and personal with the realities of our son's illness. Clothes strewn everywhere, not a stitch of them clean. Filthy dishes stacked in the sink. The refrigerator, crammed with moldy food and half-eaten scraps, looked as if a bomb had gone off inside. Dead and live roaches littered the ground, and a trail of ants would lead us to the food he'd spilled onto the floor. We began to clean. Without Heidi, I'm not sure I could have handled it. By the time we finished cleaning and had packed up his meager belongings, we were both physically and emotionally spent.

It took us a few days, but, eventually, we started to feel the weight being lifted. We were excited to have some calm in our life during Henry's three-month stint in Costa Rica. No sooner had we started feeling better than we got a phone call from a counselor at Pure Life. Henry was not happy with the discipline they instilled at the camp. It had only taken five days, but he was upset at their rules.

"Henry is not cooperating. He wants to talk to you," the head counselor told us after some preliminary greetings. He wanted us to play tough cops. "We feel that you need to lay down the law and make him stay. This is not our first rodeo, and this often happens early in their stay. We tell them that we will drop them off a mile away, and they can wait for a bus to take them into town. We wanted to call you before we let Henry talk to you, so we are all on the same page."

"That seems a little harsh," I said. "What happens if they leave? They're on their own in Costa Rica with no money?"

The counselor assured me that had rarely happened and that the few times it did, everything turned out fine, as the kids eventually came back. I was unconvinced but accepted that they were the experts. Heidi wasn't buying any of it.

"You are *not* leaving our son in Costa Rica with no money out in the jungle alone," she said incredulously. "Are you crazy? Why are you such an asshole?"

Clearly, we were not on the same page.

"Heidi, they are the experts, and they are telling us this is what we should do," I responded, though I'm not sure I believed it.

Henry called a few hours later.

"This place is a prison," he said angrily. "They even tell us when to brush our teeth. And we can't surf anytime we want. You lied to me. I want out of here. Send me a ticket home."

Our hope of peace was shattered. I spent the next few days trying to figure out what to do and talking to the counselors in Costa Rica. They assured me that this had happened before and that I shouldn't give in to Henry. They would drop Henry off at a bus stop. Once dropped off, they assumed Henry would realize he had nowhere to go and return. Clearly, they had not yet met Henry Frank Friedler. He would not come back. I didn't know what to do. I called my brother, Trost, who ran a large nonprofit addiction treatment center in Jackson, Mississippi.

Trost had a rough journey getting to the success he has today. He wasn't a good student. He was dyslexic, had ADD, and couldn't escape our intense family dynamics. Trost went to three different high schools before graduating. Overwhelmed by the chaos of his adolescence, he chose drugs as his way out. He started smoking pot at twelve and eventually got into heroin. By the time he went to college at University of Colorado in Boulder, he was a full-blown addict. My dad, after my mom died of cancer in 1983 when she was only forty-six, was dealing with his own set of problems, oblivious to Trost's. But I was not. And I was the older brother. At Christmas in 1984,

I told Trost that if he didn't get his act together, I would be forced to tell our dad. By late January of 1985, he called me from Colorado, saying he needed help. Dad had just remarried a week earlier. He and my stepmother, Pam, were on their honeymoon somewhere in Asia. I was twenty-five, in my last year in law school. While I had always experimented with drugs, unlike Trost, I knew when to stop. I had to figure out which program to put Trost in and then get him from Colorado and take him to rehab. I found a clinic in Hattiesburg, Mississippi, that would take him. I flew to Colorado and helped him to pack up. After shipping most of his stuff, Trost and I flew home. Once back, I drove him to Hattiesburg. We smoked a lot of pot on the way there, the car reminiscent of the Cheech and Chong movie with the smoke so thick you couldn't see inside the car windows. I dropped Trost off, both of us high as kites. I'm sure the counselors thought I should check in as well. I didn't give them the chance. I was right back in my car for the three-hour drive back to New Orleans.

Trost was in rehab for six months. He then went to a halfway house for another year. He's been sober ever since, over forty years. A stunning achievement and one we are all proud of. He went on to graduate from Southern Mississippi and get a degree in accounting. He got his CPA and went to work as the controller for a nonprofit rehab center. Before long, he was the CEO of the center and grew it into one of the largest nonprofit drug rehab centers in the deep South.

Trost told me I was crazy to let Henry loose in Costa Rica.

He told me Costa Rica was a dangerous place to be roaming around with no money and that I needed to get Henry home. Trost loved Henry because he was family. But also because he saw in him a kindred spirit. He believed Henry had an addiction issue and thought he knew how to help. When I refused to budge, he accused me of being too cheap to forfeit the money I had sent. He was not altogether wrong on this point. That was a lot of money to just throw away. Heidi was caught between my stubbornness and her compassion for Henry. Her compassion won, and she and Trost devised a plan. Trost sent Henry a ticket to Jackson and gave him a job in the kitchen at his facility. I pretended to be upset, but I was glad they did that. It allowed me to act as if I had set some boundaries with Henry and yet have the reassurance that he would be safe. Henry stayed with Trost and his new wife, Sarah, and her teenage daughter, Harper. I'm sure this was stressful for all of them. Henry stayed with Trost for four months. By all accounts he was well-liked at work.

It took a few months, but I started talking to Henry again. Right before Thanksgiving I suggested that he spend the holiday with us. He agreed. It seemed we would have a Thanksgiving with the entire family together.

We decided to go to Chicago for Thanksgiving to visit Heidi's family. Henry was doing better. His depression seemed less profound, and there had been no more manic episodes. He could still be moody, but being around his cousins seemed to energize him. We then took a family vacation over Christmas that also went relatively smoothly. *Relatively.* *Everything* with Henry was delicate to handle. We always felt as if we were walking on eggshells, waiting for something bad to happen. It's like watching a horror movie and not knowing when the scare is on its way. You never know when it is coming, but you know it's on its way. It's around the corner, it's in the closet, it's under the bed. And waiting for the next piece of horror was exhausting. That is the exhaustion we felt as 2015 ended. We hoped the years ahead would be better. We hoped Henry would get back on track.

chapter 13

FLORIDA

Henry was living at home again. He was moody but appeared healthy and had a job delivering food. And he was working as a tennis coach for A's and Aces, a nonprofit that provides academic assistance, life skills, and tennis instruction to the underserved kids of New Orleans. He loved working with kids. He also got a job working in a kitchen at a local restaurant. Henry enjoyed cooking, and he was good at it. Seeing that he was on a track to something, we were hopeful for him. We were still uncertain as to what was wrong with Henry. I tried to convince myself that it was nothing more than a phase, all too happy to put his struggles of the past in the rear view. So far, the only manic episode we had seen was the post-mescaline one, which allowed me to convince myself it had been a "bad trip" rather than any real disease.

Around this time Henry asked us if he could go to Santa Rosa Beach, Florida, to stay at our house for a weekend. We were reluctant to let him go alone, but Heidi and I felt it would be good for all of us. We had allowed both Kate and Patti to use the place on their own, and Henry threw that at us like a fast ball. So, we said yes and watched him drive off. And, as usual, we hoped for the best. And, as usual, that's not what we got.

Henry had been gone about two days when we got a phone call at 10 a.m. from the sheriff's office of Walton County. Henry had been picked up for loitering. The police said that he was "off." So, they took him to the nearest hospital in Fort Walton. Heidi heard me on the phone and could see in my face that something was wrong. She began to cry even before I said a word. I told her what the police had told me. She started packing an overnight bag before I had even finished, and we were in the car heading for Florida in the next fifteen minutes. The four-hour drive to Fort Walton seemed an eternity. We were silent all the way there. What was there to say? We knew of no one who had a mentally ill child. Other than Andre, we felt there was no one we could talk to. Trost, while extraordinarily helpful, still felt Henry had a drug problem. There was a stigma that surrounded mental health, and we both felt it. Fearing they wouldn't understand, we kept ourselves isolated from our friends. We unwittingly built our own little prison and put ourselves in solitary confinement.

After a very long four hours, we arrived at the hospital about 2:30. Henry had been there for twenty-four hours. He had been sedated and had slept. When he saw us, he started to cry. I tried very hard not to break down, trying to be strong. My son was in so much pain and was so utterly confused. He spoke quietly and had no idea how he had gotten to the point of being in a hospital. He agreed that he needed help and was eager to be admitted. But there was no space for him in Fort Walton.

Under Ronald Reagan's administration, we, as a country, decided that mental health wasn't as important as cutting taxes and spending. Reagan wanted mental health to be borne by the states as they saw fit. Unfortunately, many states were strapped and had neither the ability nor the interest in picking up the tab. The result was that the number of beds available for the mentally ill began to shrink. Today, when a person is walking down the street talking incoherently to strangers, the police are called. We don't treat the mentally ill, we send them to jail. To this day, whenever I pass a homeless man, I get sad thinking that could have been Henry. Without our resources and support, he would have been on the street unable to get better as he gradually slipped more and more into various states of delusion.

The doctors at the hospital in Fort Walton told us that they couldn't take him and that we'd have better luck in New Orleans. Henry agreed to go back to New Orleans with us. We checked him out and went back to our beach house, about forty-five minutes east of Fort Walton. On the way there we needed to get Henry's Honda Pilot. One problem. Henry was unable to tell us where it was. He thought he knew. But it wasn't there. He told us that he had driven somewhere, met some guys, and had done some hallucinogens with them. He thought he remembered where he had parked the car, but it was nowhere to be found. I kept pressing him, which only made him angry. The madder Henry got the more I pressed—a cycle of mutual destruction. Heidi tried to calm me down, but my temper raged. My world was falling apart, and I had no answers. "How could you not know where the car is? Come on. Just concentrate."

"I told you I left it on the road over there," Henry said, his voice becoming more and more irritated.

"Well, it's not there now. How do you explain that?" I asked, aware but unable to stop my sarcasm.

This is not a pleasant habit of mine. As I get frustrated, I tend to talk sarcastically, which everyone in the family despises.

"I don't know. Maybe the cops towed it. Call them," Henry hissed back.

So that's what I did, I called the police. They had no record of his car anywhere. After an hour searching for the car, we gave up and went back to our house. As soon as we got there, Henry jumped out of the car and took off. I doubled down on my stance, and I refused to go after him. Heidi was livid with me. In the space of a minute, I had taken Henry from a state of placidity to one of pure defiance.

"You can be such an asshole," she said. "Why do you keep escalating the situation? Can't you see the damage you do?"

Then she slammed the bedroom door, leaving me alone. I knew I had just blown it, but I was too proud and too full of ego to admit it. It's lonely knowing you're wrong and too proud to admit it. It's like digging a hole, and then getting in to dig some more. I knew I needed to go find Henry. I knew he'd be on the beach. I just had no idea where. I decided to head west and took off running. After about a mile, I saw him by the beach access at Blue Mountain, head down, walking slowly. I apologized. I told him I had gone too far and that I believed him. The car must have been stolen. I begged him to come back with me and promised that we would sort it all out. He agreed. We walked back in silence, the only sounds were the waves breaking on the beach. When we got to the house Henry went to his room and went to sleep. It turned out that the car had been exactly where Henry had thought he parked it. It had been towed by the police. It just wasn't in their system when we called.

We drove home the next day. Any goodwill we had built up with Henry was gone. He was still in his old dingy clothes, unkempt and unshaven. He slept the entire ride home. Heidi, still furious with me, spent the whole four hours purposefully engrossed in a magazine. It was a long and quiet drive. While Henry slept and Heidi fumed, I was left alone to think about all of my mistakes. I realized that Henry had been willing to get help before I bullied him about the car. Why did I feel the need to be such a jerk sometimes? Why was my temper so easily triggered? Why couldn't I see what I was doing to Henry? These were just some of the thoughts that kept me company on the road back to New Orleans.

chapter 14

WHOLE FOODS

The next few weeks were bad. Henry quit showering and wore the same clothes for days on end. He smelled bad and wouldn't look you in the eye. We would later understand these signs as the beginning of a manic phase. Over the next week, his mania morphed into psychosis. He had no car, so he would walk everywhere. It was the middle of April 2016, and the temperature was over ninety degrees—a typical hot, humid day in New Orleans—yet Henry was wearing sweatpants and a sweatshirt. His hair was long and unkempt, and he had a scraggly beard. I was on Magazine Street, grabbing some lunch near my office, when I spotted him across the street. He didn't see me, so I followed, hanging back like the CIA agents you see in the movies. He looked like any nondescript homeless guy on the street, and I almost wouldn't have recognized him. Except he was my son.

It was a confusing time for Heidi and me. Our son was drowning, and we felt helpless. We were stuck between a bunch of bad choices. As Henry had continued to get worse, we tried to persuade him to get help, to see a psychiatrist, but he refused, saying, "I'm not sick, you are." Since he was over eighteen, we had no say in the matter. American healthcare laws are so protective of the patient, it leaves little room for situations such as ours. His doctor wouldn't have been allowed to talk to us even if he had one. Which he didn't.

We were unsure of what to do, not least because Henry was yet to be diagnosed. I was still unwilling to accept the one that kept presenting itself to us: bipolar disorder. Heidi suspected it and began reading anything and everything, tireless in her ability to research the disease. She went to classes put on by the National Association of Mental Illness (NAMI). She begged me to read the books she ordered, but I refused. In my mind Henry was not bipolar. And even if he was, how could books help? I was Superman after all. I could fix this. But I wasn't and I couldn't.

In 2000, when I was forty, I decided to get a master's in counseling from Loyola University in New Orleans. As part of the curriculum, they gave us a thick book called the DSM. The DSM stands for Diagnostic and Statistical Manual of Mental Disorders. It is a reference guide for every conceivable form of mental illness. I never got my masters, but I still had my textbook. I pulled out my DSM and read through various diagnoses. Henry certainly fit the definition of bipolar to a T. Depression, check. Bouts of mania, check. Mania morphing into psychosis, check. It was impossible for me to keep my head in the sand any longer.

I trailed Henry down Magazine Street as he ambled along. He was smiling and singing loudly, oblivious to the scene he was creating. As he reached the corner of Magazine and Joseph, he wandered into the Whole Foods. Our Whole Foods in Uptown New Orleans is impressive. It's an old, converted bus barn with enormous glass windows in the front, allowing the store to be flooded with light. Through these windows I watched the show that was on full display inside. It was as if I was watching television. Or, in my case, a horror movie. Henry marched up and down the aisles, talking to anybody and nobody. As he got deeper in the store, I lost sight of him only to have him reappear in a different aisle. I could see his mouth moving, often aimed at the food along the shelves. Occasionally a person would get close enough to get his attention. While I couldn't hear him, I knew what he was saying. I had heard plenty of it—endless rants about government overreach and the ills of big business—and none of it made a ton of sense.

Fed by his recent conversion to veganism, in an attempt to regain his footing without the use of drugs, Henry always felt safe in a Whole Foods. He felt unjudged. As if the wholeness of the food transferred to the store itself. A kind of temple of the soul. But on this particular day and in this particular store, he was indeed being judged. And the verdict was not good. They asked him to leave. *Ask* being a nice way of saying the security guard escorted him out. He left peacefully, amazed that no one had been interested in his diatribe, like a small child unsure of what he had done wrong but certain that he was no longer wanted—a recurring motif in his life.

Lately, my presence seemed to set him off, so I avoided being seen. Watching Henry being escorted out, unable to help, hurt me to my core. His naïveté at what he had done wrong made it even more painful. A grown man, acting like a child, being treated as a problem. I wanted to explain to the guard that he was a good kid having a bad time. That none of this was his fault. That he was sick. But instead, I just watched as Henry left the store, his head bowed. I imagined what he must have been feeling. How harsh the world must seem. I followed him for a distance, curious what he would do next. Hoping that nothing bad would happen. But soon his head popped up and his smile returned. The wonders of a manic moment.

chapter 15

ORDER OF PROTECTIVE CUSTODY

We were left with few choices. We reached out to Cecile, the mother of a friend of Henry's from his tennis clinics, who worked for the New Orleans Police Department in the mental health unit. She was, and still is, a fierce advocate for the mentally ill and those suffering from addiction issues. She became our ally in our fight for treatment for Henry, educating us about our options. One of the few measures available to families of those suffering from mental illness is to get an Order of Protective Custody. This is a piece of paper that lasts forty-eight hours and that allows you to call the police to request they pick up a mentally ill person and take them to the psyche ward in a local hospital. The patient can then be held up to seventy-two hours for evaluation. The stays can last even longer if deemed necessary by the doctors who treat the patients. I learned that in order to get Henry the help he needed I had to go to the New Orleans Coroner's office and swear out an affidavit that Henry was a danger to himself or to others. Getting the commitment papers was the easy part. Having the nerve to use it was much harder. Heidi and I talked about it, and she asked me what I thought we should do. I've made many tough decisions in my life, but this one was the most difficult.

After getting the order, I called the police and told them I had the Order of Protective Custody. They asked me where Henry was and if he was violent. I told the dispatcher that he was at our house, and he wasn't violent. Heidi, overhearing the conversation, started crying and went upstairs to our bedroom. I heard the door shut. She couldn't handle what was coming. It was just too painful. Then, I waited in a room near the front of the house, hoping Henry would stay put. After about thirty minutes, I heard some cars entering our little street. Four police cars pulled up, each carrying two officers. The lead officer asked to see the order. He asked if Henry was still home and could I call him downstairs. Henry, who had no idea any of this was coming, came bounding downstairs, smiling like a child. When he saw all the officers, his smile vanished, replaced by a look of confusion. He looked at me with questioning eyes that melted me. I felt sick with guilt. The officer handcuffed Henry, walked him out of the house, and put him in the back of the police car. By this point it felt that everyone living in a ten-mile radius was outside watching, wondering why there were four police cars and eight cops on our tiny street. It is one of the most humiliating things that a person can go through. Why they felt the need to send so many and treat Henry like a criminal remains beyond my understanding. The fact that we have criminalized mental health in this country is inexcusable. It was a scary and humiliating process to go through for both of us. Henry was crying and scared. When I told him what

I had done, his fear and confusion turned to venom. From the open backseat of the police car, Henry shouted horrible things that cut deeply: "How could you do this to me? I hate you! You're pure evil! You're incapable of love and should never have had kids!"

The last one stung. In his mind, he wasn't sick. I was torturing him for no reason. And it hurt because some part of me felt that way as well. I didn't want this to be happening. I didn't want him in the back of a police car handcuffed and in tears. I just wanted my sweet Henry back. Having been cornered into using this broken system made me feel dirty. It was a horrible choice between two horrible options. To have him view it as a betrayal cut even deeper. I wasn't caught between a rock and a hard place. I was between a mountain and hell.

I was told they were taking him to University Hospital's emergency room and to meet them there. I went upstairs to tell Heidi. She was in our bedroom with the door still closed. When I opened it, I saw her lying on the bed crying. She looked at me with her red, moist eyes and made me feel even worse. She knew we did what we had to, but I felt so alone. She couldn't go to the hospital, couldn't even get off the bed. Paralyzed by the trauma of our situation, she asked me if I would go to the hospital without her. It was all a bridge too far for her. I lay down next to her and held her hand as we both cried for another minute. Then I wiped my eyes, got out of bed, and left for the hospital.

When I got to the emergency room, no one could tell me anything other than Henry was there. Fortunately, I recognized one of the nurses from my gym, who said he would check on Henry. He told me to wait in the coffee shop, and he would find out more. After nearly an hour and three cups of coffee, I saw him looking for me. He told me that they were holding Henry, waiting for a bed to open. Twenty years after Reagan had cut back federal spending on mental health, Bobby Jindal became Governor of Louisiana. His administration further decimated Louisiana's mental health services. As Governor he pushed through cuts that reduced the number of psychiatric hospital beds in New Orleans by about 20%—hence the difficulty in finding a bed for Henry. The first bed the doctors found was at Ochsner Hospital, twenty minutes away in Jefferson Parish. We were lucky. We heard stories of patients being sent as far as three hours away. I watched as Henry was put in the ambulance on his way to Ochsner.

By the next day, Heidi had recovered and desperately wanted to see Henry. This was our first visit to a psychiatric ward. It would not be our last. In order to see Henry, we had to first go through security. We had to remove our keys, wallets, and phones and leave them with the officer. We were then buzzed through a set of steel doors into the psych ward. It's a place unlike any other hospital wing. There was a large, sterile common space. There were few windows, with little natural light. The harsh fluorescent lights made it even bleaker. The other patients looked drugged and seemed to move in slow motion. Think "One Flew Over the Cuckoo's Nest." There were plenty of places to sit, but all lacked privacy. A TV was blasting away with no one watching. We saw Henry seated at the far end of the room, looking down. As we approached, he looked up at us, barely acknowledging our presence. He was in hospital clothes, a green top with blue cotton pants tied at the waist. He had on hospital slippers that were too big for him. He was no longer in a psychotic state. The medicine they were giving him worked. But he was *pissed*. "Why did you do this to me? You're the devil. This place is jail. Get me out," he ranted at us.

"Henry, what else could we do?" Heidi asked. "You were out of control and talking nonsense. We were scared. We're just trying to help."

"You think this is helping me? Surrounded by crazy people?" Henry asked, unaware of the irony. "Either help me get out *now* or leave."

"Henry, we have no control at this point. It's up to the doctors now," I said, realizing how lame that sounded.

"Well then, I'm here for a while. They're paid to keep me here," Henry said with resignation. "Just go. I don't want you here."

Even in a semi-manic state, Henry was right. The system is set up to keep beds full. Hospitals make good money on psychiatric patients. However, due to the shortage of beds, patients get cycled through faster. They would release him once he was out of his manic state. Henry is smart, and he quickly understood this. He settled down and did whatever they asked. He took his medication and slept at night. After four days he was well enough to be released, telling his doctors he would continue taking his prescribed medications.

On May 3, Henry called us to let us know he was being released later that day. Heidi and I both went to the hospital to pick him up. Henry was released into our custody with two bottles of pills and instructions on taking them. As soon as we got in the car, Henry's anger spewed out in full force: "I hope you're happy with yourselves. You disgust me. You say you love me then you send me to a place like this? You tell me I have a problem? Clearly you two are the ones with a problem. Take me home and leave me alone and DO NOT ASK ME ABOUT MY MEDICATION. It is none of your business."

"Henry, do you think we like this?" I said, in a low tone. "We felt we had no choice. You were out of control, and we needed to get you to calm down. This was not our first choice."

"Whatever," he spat contemptuously. "Just bring me home."

We soon established a détente where we co-existed. He stayed away from us, eating alone and spending most of his time in his room. We tried our best to give him time to get better. After a week we could tell he was not taking his meds. He wouldn't sleep. He wouldn't shower. He barely ate. At twenty-three, he was 5'11" but weighed 145 tops. He wore the same dirty clothes that hung off his slight figure for days on end. He would leave the house to just wander around. He had no car, so he did plenty of walking. We worried and kept hoping he would sleep and improve. We didn't want to send him back to the hospital. But he just kept getting worse. The mania turned into psychosis again, and we soon felt we were out of options.

Kate, home from college, was witnessing this behavior for the first time. She had never seen Henry in a psychotic state. Seeing her energy twin so wound up terrified her. The three of us had long talks about his condition. We spent days hoping he would snap out of his mania. I'm not a very religious person, yet I prayed for a miracle. Unanswered prayers. Finally, Heidi and I agreed we should return to the New Orleans Coroner's office to get another Order of Protective Custody. Heidi and I now knew the drill and the calamity that it caused. We knew that Henry would be irate. We knew that he would hate us for doing it. We long ago gave up the notion that we were Henry's friend. It was time to be his parents. Yet, having to parent like this remains one of the hardest things we have ever had to do. We would have done anything to avoid calling the police and starting the process all over again. Heidi wanted me to make the phone call. She just couldn't do it. It was too painful. Kate took off, so she could avoid the inevitable.

Once Kate was gone and Heidi was in our bedroom with the door shut, I made the call. Henry was once again caught totally unaware. This time he knew the drill, staring at me with cold hard eyes, incredulous that I had done it again. After Henry was placed in the police car, I asked the officer if he could take Henry directly to Ochsner this time as I knew the doctors there knew him. There were no beds at Ochsner. The closest available bed was at a psychiatric facility called Seaside in Baton Rouge, seventy miles away. That's where he was sent, and, by the time we found out where he was, it was too late to visit. We weren't allowed to visit until the next day. We made plans to go, and Kate insisted on coming.

Having three kids so close in age can be a lot of work. Kate and Henry always had a great relationship. There was the usual drama, of course. But they had an unbreakable bond. He was close to Patti too, who was three years older. They were all very different kids. Henry was cocky and competitive. Patti was not. They both knew how to push each other's buttons and would do it just for sport. But while they would be screaming one minute over who gets to watch what show, they would be watching the same show ten minutes later, laughing at the same things, shoulders touching. No matter how hard they fought, all my kids had each other's back. There was a deep love between them, a love only siblings know. Often, Patti and Henry were co-conspirators in Henry's impressive playbook on how to torture Kate. Once when Henry was ten and Patti was thirteen, I was driving them home from soccer practice. I could hear whispering and giggling in the back. They were clearly concocting something. When they got home, they ran upstairs and three minutes later I heard Kate screaming. I ran upstairs to see Henry holding Kate down while Patti was rubbing her smelly shin guards in Kate's face. Clearly this had been the grand plan they had been discussing. When Patti went off to college, they didn't talk as much. But when we were all together for vacations and holidays, Heidi and I could see how much our kids loved each other.

When Henry's disease took over, Patti was living in New York, and her distance kept her out of the fray. But Kate became even closer to Henry. She was always there when he needed her. Kate was one of Henry's biggest defenders. Because they were only a year apart, they had many of the same friends. Kate watched some of those friends distance themselves from Henry, which was understandable, given his erratic behavior. She did what she could to keep them all connected, but it was hard. As Henry got sicker, more people washed their hands of him and gave up. Kate never did. She always included Henry in her plans—and lost some friends in doing so. I worried that she was carrying more responsibility than was healthy for her. She was young, and this wasn't her burden to shoulder. Yet, she took it on like it was her duty. Kate was Henry's energy twin, and she took it upon herself to look after him, no matter how hard it got.

And now she wanted to go to Baton Rouge with us to visit Henry. We were conflicted. We thought Henry might enjoy seeing Kate, but, at the same time, we were worried that Kate would be overwhelmed. Or that she might catch some not so friendly fire. She had never been to a psychiatric ward, and we knew it would be rough. Heidi felt strongly that Henry would appreciate it, and I agreed. We told her she could come.

We arrived at Seaside Hospital early the following afternoon. It was a small, concrete building surrounded by a concrete parking lot. Too small to be a hospital. It looked more like a dentist's office. The inside was no better. The ceilings were eight feet and the whole place reeked of neglect. We checked in with the receptionist, left all our personal items with the security guard, walked through some locked doors, and entered a large common space. Like at Ochsner there was the same TV blasting with no one watching. The walls were a mustard yellow, peeling and unable to hide the dirt. Once again, there were plenty of seats and no privacy. The other patients were either sitting comatose in a chair or walking around mumbling to themselves. I looked over at Kate. She looked startled. Her eyes were wide and her mouth a little open.

We saw Henry about the same time he saw us. He was happy to see Kate; he felt he had an ally in her. But he was furious with Heidi and me. He complained at length about how miserable the place was. And it was. I could see Kate looking around, still trying to process what she was seeing. Henry began talking directly to her as if we weren't even there.

"Kate," he began. "You need to get me out of here. Mom and Dad are evil to put me in here. Will you help?"

Kate was having a tough time. It was just too much. Her eyes started to water, and I could see she was close to losing it. She quickly made some excuse to leave and went to wait outside. She later told me that by the time she'd reached the car she couldn't hold back the tears. Leaning against the car for support, Kate sobbed, unnerved by what she had seen. A woman from across the parking lot saw the whole scene and approached her. As she made her way over, Kate tried to straighten up and regain her composure. The woman, an African-American in her mid-forties, asked gently if she had a loved one inside. Between sobs Kate told her that her brother was inside. The woman nodded and said her sister was in there, too. She asked if she could give Kate a hug. Kate opened her arms and walked into the embrace of this stranger and melted into her arms. This woman she didn't know, giving her the empathy and understanding she desperately needed. Often, during our years of dealing with Henry's illness, a hug was all we needed. To feel seen in our struggle and consoled even for a moment. But in our fight with Henry's disease, such acts of generosity were rare.

Meanwhile, Heidi and I were inside. And there were no hugs. Caught between the deep sadness of this place and the despair of our son, we once again endured Henry's onslaught. Henry wanted out. He knew they could only keep him for seventy-two hours. After that it would be up to the doctors. Henry hated that they had that power over him. He ranted against the place and especially against the doctor in charge. The head psychiatrist was a no-bullshit guy who Henry despised. We couldn't talk to the doctor without Henry's written permission. Incredibly, without this waiver we'd be unable to talk to any of his doctors. And we wouldn't be able to be a part of any treatment plan. Henry signed the waiver. He just wanted out.

The doctor had time for us and led us into his office. He told us that Henry was still manic and needed more time. He was not ready to give us a diagnosis, but, on our next visit, he would have more information. He was generous with his time but had to cut us short: we didn't have an appointment and he was late for a meeting.

Henry was waiting, hoping that he would be leaving with us. We told him that he had to stay. He was pissed. He told us to leave and to not come back until he could come home. We left and found Kate leaning against the car. It was a long, quiet ride back to New Orleans.

With Henry seventy miles away in Baton Rouge, a twenty-minute visit with him took about four hours round trip. And that assumed he would even be *willing* to see us. Yet, we had no choice. Our son was in a psych ward, in a strange city, and he needed to know we cared. Heidi and I planned to go back to Seaside the next day. As we were getting ready for the ride up, we got a phone call from Seaside. Before we had time to worry, the nurse on the other end said, "Everything is fine." What? I assumed it was until I got this call. Now, I was a little less sure.

She went on, "Henry was involved in a slight altercation. He's fine. We are just taking him to the hospital for a checkup. He is right here. I'll put him on."

"Dad, I'm fine," he said with an "I-told-you-so" tone. "They're taking me to the emergency room just to be safe. I have to go." And he hung up.

This raised our guilt meters considerably. Henry had been in the wrong place at the wrong time. Caught between two patients fighting over the TV, Henry took a hard left to the head. Apparently, they do watch those TVs. For Heidi and me, this was yet another glimpse into the terrible world of mental hospitals, chaotic places filled with too many sick people, some of whom had been sick for decades. Henry, a relative newbie to this world, seemed to have his shit together compared to these lifers. With bipolar disorder and other psychotic disorders, the longer the illness goes untreated, the worse the patient becomes. Years of psychotic breaks take their toll, which was why Heidi and I were desperate to get Henry the treatment he needed right away. We just didn't yet know what that treatment was.

We drove up the next day, but Henry refused to see us. I would like to think he appreciated the effort. For the next few days, he would call us but not allow us to visit. He wanted out and kept pressing the doctors. The Seaside doctors held Henry for three more days, giving him time to recover from his psychotic break. A week after being admitted, we went to Baton Rouge to pick him up.

Before he was released, we sat down with the head doctor, who told us that he believed Henry had bipolar disorder. This was the first time that a doctor had given us that diagnosis. The doctor was incredibly generous with his time and answered every question we had. He explained bipolar disorder and its treatment. Heidi was willing to accept the diagnosis. It meant she could begin planning a course of action. But I was not. I fought it the same way I fight everything that frustrates me. Relentlessly. I was a man who made his living by making people accept and see clearly the realities of their lives. Yet, I refused to accept my own. I was scared to death of that diagnosis. So, I fought it. I thought that if I willed it to not be true, then it wouldn't be true.

We all agreed that Henry should go to a facility that could provide long-term treatment. And while I say we all agreed, I mean Heidi, the doctor, and me. Henry had not yet consented, and therein lay the problem. Since he was over eighteen, without his cooperation, we had no say in the matter.

The doctor then called Henry in with us. He told Henry that he was being released on the condition he would take his medication and get a doctor who could monitor his progress. He suggested a few months at a longer care facility. Henry was smart enough to know that if he just said yes to everything, they would release him. We gathered his stuff and checked him out.

It took two minutes in the car on the ride back to New Orleans for him to reverse course. And I think I'm being generous. He began by berating Heidi and me for calling the police in the first place. He then went after the legal system. Next up, the hospital system. Finally, he took on big pharma. As to that last point it was hard to argue with him. Turn on your TV, and most of the ads you will see are for drugs. Drugs for diabetes, drugs for eczema, drugs for HIV. There are plenty for bipolar disorder, as well. The ads make it sound as if, with a few pills, bipolar disorder is manageable, like diabetes or eczema. And while the drugs do help many, they have their terrible side effects—things like weight gain; akathisia, a form of restlessness; and tardive dyskinesia, uncontrollable move-ments of the jaw, lips, and tongue—making it even harder to go through life unnoticed. It's like exchanging one monstrous disease for several slightly less nasty ones. No matter. Henry didn't want to be medicated, so drugs were a nonstarter.

When we got home, he went up to his room and shut the door. At least we knew he was not manic anymore. Unfortunately, he was depressed again. The brutal nature of the disease is that it sends you back and forth between depres-sion and mania like an out-of-control roller coaster, taking both rider and bystander on an awful and disorienting ride. It devastated both Heidi and me to see our son so sick. And it frustrated and angered me that I was helpless to help. We started looking for long-term clinics close to New Orleans that would take Henry.

Most of the places we explored treated addiction and men-tal health as if they were the same thing. To be sure, many mentally ill patients abuse drugs. But not all drug abusers have a mental illness. We knew that Henry's main problem was his bipolar disorder. It was vital that we found a place that primar-ily treated mental illness. We also needed a place that Henry would agree to go to. We weren't having much luck, so we called our friend Cecile, who had told us about the Protective Custody Order. She gave us the name of a clinic in North Carolina, CooperRiis. CooperRiis specialized in mental health issues. We called, and CooperRiis said they would take Henry if he wanted to go. Getting Henry to agree was a whole other story.

chapter 16

ESCAPE FROM COOPERRIIS

Henry had been home about a week, and the house was rife with tension. He was moody and depressed, staying holed up in his room. When he emerged, he ignored us. In that rare moment when he would talk to us, Heidi asked him if he would look at a clinic we thought he might like. He looked at the CooperRiis website and admitted it seemed like a nice place. It was in rural North Carolina, and Henry liked that they had their own farm and tennis courts. But there was an insurmountable problem: Henry refused to admit that he was sick. We were at a stalemate. Henry refused to go to CooperRiis, and there was nothing we could do to make him go.

Heidi called Cecile for advice. Her son Chris was familiar with Cooper Riis. Chris and Henry were the same age, had grown up playing tennis together, and knew each other well. She said she would ask Chris to talk to Henry. Chris called Henry, and they made plans to play tennis. Whatever Chris said to Henry worked, because he came home, sweating and smiling, and said he would go to CooperRiis. He even said Chris would drive him up there. We called CooperRiis, and they told us there would be a room available in three days. Chris, with Cecile's blessing, agreed to drive Henry there—another act of kindness that overwhelmed us. Chris' generosity and care for Henry was a tribute to both Cecile and Chris. In a sea of loneliness, they invited us into their lifeboat.

Still, Heidi and I felt we couldn't let Chris handle this burden alone. What if Henry refused to check in once they got there? I had a meeting in New Orleans I couldn't miss, so Heidi agreed to drive up as well. Henry refused to let Heidi drive with them. Not wanting to press our luck, Heidi agreed to go in a separate car, an eight-hour drive that she made alone. Heidi, of course, never complained, though I know how hard it was for her to do this alone. She wanted her son better and would do anything for that end. Thinking back, I find it hard to understand how I let Heidi shoulder this burden alone. How hard that eight-hour drive must have been, with nothing to do but worry about Henry. What meeting of mine could have been so important?

The boys left before Heidi and got a hotel near CooperRiis. Chris called me when they got there and said Henry was doing well. Tomorrow, they would begin the admission process, where Henry would have interviews in the morning. Heidi would arrive in the afternoon to discuss his admission. If all went well, he would check in that afternoon, and Heidi would drive right back home. Heidi did not arrive until after dark and checked into a different hotel. She called me from the hotel, exhausted from her drive and anxious about the next day. I told her about my conversation with Chris and tried to cheer her up, but I could feel her deepening anxiety.

The next morning, she met Chris and Henry at CooperRiis for Henry's first meetings with a therapist. By lunchtime Henry was no longer willing to go. We had no idea why he had changed his mind. Maybe the therapist reminded him of his father or some other authority figure. Who knows? Heidi pleaded with Henry to no avail. She left dejected and deflated for the long drive back to New Orleans. Chris, meanwhile, took Henry back to the hotel to check out. During that time, he somehow convinced Henry to give CooperRiis a try. Heidi was an hour into her return trip when Chris called to tell her Henry had changed his mind and was being admitted. She was happy but exhausted from all the back and forth. From the roller coaster of Henry. She called me in tears. I convinced her to stop at our place in Florida and spend a few days at the beach, for some much-needed time alone. She agreed and changed her route to stop at Florida. By now it was getting dark, and she had to take a series of two-lane roads through the back country of Alabama. I stayed on the phone with her for an hour, keeping her company and making sure she made no wrong turns. It was exhausting for both of us. When Heidi finally made it to our place in Florida it was 10 p.m., and she had nothing left. She climbed into bed and slept until 10 the next morning. On the phone the next morning, she said she felt better and wanted to spend another few days at the beach. This made me happy. I knew she needed the time alone.

With Henry at CooperRiis. I felt I could finally relax. I was wrong. After only six days, Henry had another psychotic episode. The clinic called me that afternoon to tell me what had happened. The police had been called, and Henry had been fished out of the pond on the campus which he had jumped into in order to "escape." He was taken directly to a hospital in town and would be held there until he could be safely released back to CooperRiis. Henry stayed in that hospital for seven days. Once he was sedated and given antipsychotic medication, his state improved. We were able to talk to him, but he was bored and restless. No one from CooperRiis came to visit him while he was in the hospital. This did not sit well with either of us, but particularly Henry. He felt that the people at the treatment center didn't care about him. That put an end to any willingness he might have had to stay on in the program.

When Henry returned to the treatment center, he called us immediately and told us he wanted to leave. Heidi and I were getting ready for our summer vacation in Michigan. We were exhausted and desperately needed a break. We had long conversations about what to do and decided that Henry needed to stay put. He needed help to get better, and we could no longer do it ourselves. In concert with Heidi, I told him that if he left early, he would be on his own. This was a big step for Heidi. For years, she had been unwilling to practice any sort of "tough love" on Henry.

Even as I write the words, I am struck by how ridiculous the notion of tough love is. These are lose-lose situations in which no one is happy. As parents we loved our kids uncon- ditionally. But the exhaustion and despair of dealing nonstop with a mentally ill child wore us down. We weren't ready to lose Henry, but we were losing the strength to deal with his demons. And we were running out of options to address his mental illness. So, we resorted to tough love. It's like being asked to watch a child drown and hope they will eventually pop up and swim to shore—few parents can sit back and do this. But too tired and too confused to do anything else, we were willing to take our chances. We were willing to allow Henry to make his own mistakes. While I had arrived at that place earlier, the car ride and dealing with Henry alone had been the straw that broke Heidi's back. After the apartments, Costa Rica, the fights at home, the inpatient psyche wards, she was completely exhausted. We both were.

We had numerous phone calls with both Henry and CooperRiis. We let Henry know that he needed to stay and that if he left, he would be on his own. Undeterred by our threats, Henry left CooperRiis and took a bus to Destin, Florida. I got a tracking device that I could install in his car. I'd had his car towed to the offices of the rental company that oversaw our beach house a few days after the Florida incident. I sent them the tracking device, and they put it in his car the day he got to Florida. He had no access to our place, as it was rented. At this point, we cut him off financially. Tough love.

Henry, clearly delusional, was determined to live out of his car until he got a job. And that's what he did. He began living in his car with no job, no money, and no prospects. But it was June. June in the panhandle of Florida. And after two days of extreme heat, he called me. As difficult as it was to say this, Heidi and I told him he had made his choice, and he needed to live with the consequences. We would pay for him to go back to CooperRiis. But we would pay for nothing else.

For all my toughness and bravado with Heidi, I found it difficult to let Henry suffer. It's not easy to see your child hurting. I consulted Trost often for advice. And though Trost was the one who bailed Henry out of Costa Rica, he would constantly ride me for "enabling" Henry. I believe he still thought Henry had an addiction issue. We all see the world through our own prism, and Trost's was the world of addiction. Enabling is a big word in the addict community, and, while I agreed with him in principle, it just felt wrong to be so tough on a kid who was struggling with mental illness. I wasn't sure where to draw the line between enabling and helping. Or if it even matters. Nothing will work unless the patient is ready to accept help. As long as they feel they don't have a problem, it is pointless to offer a solution. If Henry refused treatment and medication, there was little we could do for him. Yet, it's much easier to say that than to actually look the other way. Knowing he was out there fending for himself, alone and living in his car with no money, was brutal. I wanted to help Henry, but in a way he would not detect. I had drawn my line in the sand and felt that in order to maintain my believability, I couldn't fold. I was playing a game of chicken and didn't want to let Henry win. He needed to truly believe we had cut him off. I wanted him to know I was serious. I also wanted him safe. So, I cheated.

chapter 17

I called Trost and told him what was going on with Henry. We devised a plan. It felt devious. Trost would reach out to Henry and offer him a place to stay in Jackson and a job in the cafeteria at the clinic. I agreed to donate to the clinic an amount that would more than offset the extra cost. A win-win for Heidi and me. Henry, who was probably hungry and tired of living in his car, accepted the offer and drove immediately to Jackson, having no idea that his dad's donation was behind his new living arrangement.

Henry settled in and quickly fell into his new life. A kindred spirit, he was liked by the other workers. Henry always found it easy to make friends, and Jackson was no exception. All was good and Heidi and I could relax a little knowing he was under the watchful eye of my brother.

It was also time for our favorite week of the year.

Every summer, during the last week in June, we would head to the Watervale Inn in upper Michigan for our family vacation. To call it a resort is generous at best. Though for us, it is as spectacular as any five-star spa. The same family has owned and operated it for over a hundred years. The women of the family are in charge. When Heidi was a kid, Vera ran it. When I started going, Vera's daughter Dori ran it. And now Dori's daughter, Jennie, runs it with an iron fist and a sweet smile. Heidi's family has been going for over fifty years. Every week the same group of people inhabits the place. In our over thirty years of going, we had become quite close to the other families with whom we shared our week. Watervale is a place that time has forgotten. There are no televisions, and the only available phone is behind the counter at the inn. In the days before cell phones, that one phone was the only way you could be reached. Watervale is peace on earth. An actual escape from the real world. It is hard to be found in a place that time forgot.

Watervale consists of several small cottages and the inn. The cottages are simple, each with its own name and particular charm. When our family first started going, we would always stay at the Ursula, one door down from the inn. The Margret was a larger cottage, closer to Lake Michigan, with its own small beach on the little lake. We coveted the Margret, but someone else had it. The only way to get it would be if a family stopped coming—which would never happen. Yet, one summer we got a call from Jennie. The Margret was now available, and did we want it? I didn't even have to consult my family.

"Yes, please, we want it."

To this day it's where we stay during our week there. I imagine we'll still be there twenty years from now.

They serve breakfast between 8 to 10 a.m. and dinner in two seatings. We always went to the late seating at 7:15 p.m. When the bell rang, you knew it was time. The little kids would all fight over who got to ring the bell. When the kids were young, we sat in the main dining room at a large table for twelve. There were the five of us, Heidi's brother Chip, his wife Jenny, and our three nephews, plus Heidi's parents, Chuck and Lori. As the kids got older, we were given the west porch. This was a major upgrade. Where Watervale royalty sat. At least that was how we felt. We take over the whole porch now, with cousins and aunts and uncles. Every night it's a mini family reunion. You have the same servers for every meal, and it's always the college-age son or daughter of a family who goes to Watervale. The server's job is a plumb assignment. Tips are good. Since they serve the same families for the entire week, it becomes a friendship. They know your name, your kids' names, and you know theirs. If you don't know your server, the first question you ask is, "What week does your family come?" Ever since they were little, my girls have wanted to be waitresses there. You have to have finished your freshman year of college before you can apply. Both my girls did it for the full three years. Henry had no desire.

One of our favorite things was the Baldy hike. Baldy is a sand dune about 300 yards above Lake Michigan. The only way to get there is through the woods. You hike down a road and then start the trail that goes up and down like those settings on a treadmill. After about one mile you hit "Heart Attack Hill," a sandy, uphill climb. When you reach the top, you emerge from the woods and into a field of blue and yellow wildflowers and long dune grass. Then it's another quarter mile or so through sand, flowers, and grass until you turn a corner and see Lake Michigan gleaming blue and stretching forever. Then the fun part. You run down the dune, heels kicking up, leaning backwards for balance, as gravity does its thing. After cleaning the sand out of your shoes, you walk back along Lake Michigan, whose water is cold even in late June. The hike back is usually done with your eyes down, searching for Petoskey stones, round rocks composed of fossilized coral. Heidi was a savant at finding them. I was not.

Henry used to love to run the Baldy hike. He would challenge me, and, like a fool, I would accept. I did my best to keep up, but by the time he was twelve, it was a lost cause. Once, he got so far ahead of me I lost sight of him. As I was running back along the beach, gasping for air, I saw some friends and asked if they had seen Henry. Yes, they said, about twenty minutes ago, and asked if the grey in my beard was weighing me down.

Watervale has two tennis courts and not many tennis players. There was no one there who was as good as I was, much less Henry. We would hit almost every day. Shirts off, sweating after a few minutes of cross-court forehands. Heidi *loved* these moments. She didn't get to see Henry hit as much as she would have liked. At Watervale she got to see him every day. Soon word got out that we were hitting and before too long a small crowd began to form. I would like to think they came to watch me. I knew, of course, they came to watch Henry.

But Henry was on his way to Jackson. This would be the first year that we would not be there with the whole family.

The drive from Chicago to Watervale is about five hours. When you leave Route 31 for county highway M22, you know you're close. You go through green, rolling hills and then through the towns of Onekama, then Arcadia, and, as you come down from a large hill, you see Blaine cemetery on the right and know you're there. At the cemetery you take a left, down Watervale Road. Taking that left, I grabbed Heidi's hand for reassurance. We were both crying. I was unprepared for these emotions. It was a clear sign that life was out of order. Henry loved Watervale as much as we did, maybe even more so, yet he wasn't there. His absence was a constant reminder that things were broken. Our family was hurting, and even Watervale could not put us back together again. It was tough to be there without Henry, and, while this would be the first time, it would not be the last. Each time that week I passed the tennis courts, I thought of Henry. Every Baldy hike. Every meal. He was not there, his absence hovering over everything. Our friends would ask, and sometimes we would tell them. Having to relive all that had transpired made the week even tougher. We were tired of the drama, and, while Watervale had always been a perfect place to escape, without Henry, Watervale just didn't feel like Watervale.

chapter 18

MILLSAPS

We returned from Michigan as Henry settled into his new life in Jackson. Like a spy behind enemy lines, Trost kept us posted. Three months ago, Henry had been in a psychiatric ward. Now, he seemed fine. The thing about bipolar disorder is its terrible ups and downs. Lately, all we had been experiencing were the downs. We were about to go on a great ride up.

Trost's house was a short walk to Millsaps College, a small liberal arts school in the heart of Jackson. Henry would wander over to the campus often, drawn, of course, to the tennis courts. He watched the tennis coach hitting balls with players during that July. After a few days of watching, Henry got an itch and walked over to talk with the coach. Henry told him that he had been a highly ranked Southern tennis player and asked if there was room on the team for him. The coach hit with Henry. Even though Henry had not hit a tennis ball in over a year, it didn't take long for the coach to see the talent he had before him. He asked if Henry would like to go to Millsaps. It had a total enrollment of only 750 kids and was a member of the NCAA Division III in the Southern Athletic Conference with other small schools like Rhodes, Sewanee, and Centre College. Henry wanted more from life and knew that he needed to do something other than work in a kitchen. He also knew I would pay for college. Henry was twenty-three and had only three semesters of college credit, yet the coach had little problem getting him admitted. His grades and board scores were so good they offered him a scholarship, making his tuition very reasonable. Heidi and I were beside ourselves. This was the kind of college experience we had always hoped for Henry.

College had been a great experience for both of us, full of friends and funny stories. Heidi has kept up with her college friends, the same core group of eight women who all went to St. Lawrence University together. Other than one whose husband died and one who died of ALS, they are all still alive and married. They get together at least once a year at each other's homes, and the husbands are asked to get scarce for the weekend. We've hosted one in New Orleans and one at our place in Florida. I have always envied Heidi's friendships as I have few like hers. It is a tribute to Heidi that she has been a part of such an exceptional group for such a long time. This was what she always wanted for Henry.

Millsaps, while smaller than the schools we attended, had that college feel we both remembered. Over the past several years, we had been worn down by the chaos that had engulfed our family. Like an oasis appearing to a parched man trapped in a lonely desert, Millsaps materialized. For the first time in a long time, we were hopeful.

Moving him into his dorm was a delight, the experience we had been waiting for. He was excited and surrounded by new friends. He was playing tennis and smiling constantly, unable to contain his happiness with his new life. Yet, he was unwilling to allow us to share in that happiness—payback for all of our "sins." He blamed us for his hospitalizations. His feelings of betrayal ran deep, and there was a piece of me that understood. What we had done, while necessary, was tough on him. And while Henry couldn't see it, we had always done what we thought was the right thing. But in his eyes, we were the enemy. Deep down, I suspected he loved us. Sometimes it was very deep down.

Henry would not let us come to any of his matches. We continuously asked, and he continuously refused. Heidi and I respected his wishes and stayed away. I imagine his teammates and their parents wondered why we were not around. By the end of the season, Henry relented and invited us up for a weekend. They had a match on Saturday and one Sunday. Watching him play those matches, watching him interact with his teammates, was enough for us.

Henry took to Millsaps wholeheartedly. It was as if he had never been sick. He excelled in his classes and loved being part of the tennis team. A college tennis match consists of three doubles teams and six singles players. Your best player plays #1, the next best plays #2, and so forth. Henry, other than playing #1 and #2 a couple of times, played mostly #3 on the team where he only lost one match. He also played #2 doubles where he and his partner had a winning record. Henry was thriving on the court and in the classroom, where he was majoring in education. After his first year, he was an Academic All-American in his conference. He also joined the fraternity that many of his teammates were in.

Henry did all this unmedicated. This was hard for me to understand. On the one hand, I am being told that my son has bipolar disorder and will need medication for the rest of his life; on the other hand, here he was, unmedicated and thriving. I have subsequently learned that this is another complexity of this insidious disease. It's always hiding around the corner, waiting for the right moment to pounce.

Henry finished his year and had enough credits to start his junior year. He joined us that summer at Watervale. Life was looking up. Henry had always wanted to spend a semester in Europe, and, given his recent accomplishments, we were sure he had earned it. He needed to go during the fall as tennis season was in the spring. Since they practiced year-round, his coach was reluctant to lose him but allowed him to go. We got all of the paperwork together that summer and off he went to Seville, Spain. Henry had taken years of Spanish and was rather good at speaking it. He thought Spain would be a perfect place for him to see Europe and further improve his Spanish.

It was a nervous four months. While we were pleased with Henry's progress, we were anxious about him being in Europe with little supervision. I can't really say why, but I could sense that Henry was slipping again. Maybe it was the lack of structure, or maybe it was just muscle memory. Either way, I had an uneasy feeling about his time in Spain. We knew he was traveling because we could track him via his credit card spending. He was so far away, and the time zones were so different that we did not talk much. I'm sure Henry enjoyed this, but, for us, it was torture. Especially for me. It is hard to control things on a different continent. If he made any friends, he never mentioned it. He didn't complain much, and when he did it was about his grades, which he felt should be better.

When it was time to come back, I had nightmares that he would refuse. Now adjusted to an independent life over in Europe, I could see him going dark and disappearing forever. Those were the kind of mind games I was playing with myself. I scheduled his flights back to New Orleans. To get him home, he had to change planes twice in Europe. The first time in Madrid, the second in Amsterdam, two spots that I knew he loved. Two points from which he could disappear forever. My brain went into overdrive. What would happen if he had a manic episode over in Europe, or on the day of his flight? What would we do then? Would I have to go to Europe and search for him, like in a Liam Neeson movie? So, when Henry got off the plane in New Orleans, I was relieved.

We had planned a family vacation that Christmas of 2018. We were leaving just a few days after he returned for Lapland in northern Finland to chase the Northern Lights. We would spend Christmas there, New Years in Copenhagen, then head home. By the time Henry was back in New Orleans, he did not want to go with us. In retrospect I should have let him stay home. I could tell he was depressed, but I love it when we are all together. Family vacations are what I live and work for. Not having Henry come with us felt wrong. It was a terrible time in the run up to that vacation, as Heidi was inclined to let him stay home. I bullied both of them until Henry agreed to come with us.

Lapland was cold. Very cold. The high never got much above zero degrees. The sun never rose. It was dusk from 11 a.m. to about 2 p.m., and, for the rest of the day, it was dark. The wrong place for a depressed kid, dark and cold with no sunlight. He stayed at the hotel most days as we did things like reindeer rides and dog sleds, where we froze and wished we were indoors with Henry. We were lucky enough to see the Northern Lights twice. They were beautiful, and Henry was as excited as the rest of us. But between Henry's depression and Heidi still being angry at me for making him come, it was not a great few days. Unlike the weather, Heidi eventually thawed. Henry rallied as well, and we ended up having some memorable moments.

We left Finland the day after Christmas and headed to Copenhagen, where it was a balmy thirty degrees. We were staying at the Tivoli Gardens hotel, which is connected to the amusement park, so we had free admission each night. The girls loved it and rode many of the rides. They especially loved the roller coaster and begged me to go with them. I had already been on a three-year ride of my own, so I chose not to go. Their smiles and screams warmed me even in the cold. Henry, however, found a poker room and spent little time with us. He would join us for dinner, but after each meal he went off by himself to play poker, which had become a big part of Henry's life ever since Oregon. He was good at it and won more than he lost.

Upon our return to New Orleans, I felt that Henry was slipping into mania. Heidi felt it, too. He was doing so well, and the chaos had finally disappeared. We were not eager for it to return. I wanted to believe that the signs I was seeing—lack of sleep, lack of showering, fast talking—were in my head. I wanted to believe that, since he had done so well at Millsaps, going back to Millsaps was all he needed. Heidi felt the same way. Henry was, in fact, eager to get back to school, which we took as a good sign. I hoped I was just being overly sensitive and that being back at Millsaps was the answer. These were just a few of the other lies I told myself. I was doing exactly what I recommended that my clients avoid. I was ignoring reality. I was a man seeing a mirage, not an oasis.

chapter 19

LEAVING MILLSAPS

Henry drove back to Millsaps on January 7, 2018, to start the second semester of his junior year. He was twenty-five years old. A few weeks after being back, the tennis coach called us to ask if we had noticed anything "off" about Henry. The coach said he was not acting like himself. He added that Henry had been "inappropriate" with the team's yoga instructor and that his class attendance was not good.

When you have a loved one with a mental illness, you learn to walk a tightrope. Straddling the line between respecting the privacy of the individual and summoning the help they may need in a crisis, we had chosen to protect Henry's privacy. He'd been doing well at Millsaps, so we never told anyone about his condition. After the phone conversation with the coach, his secret would be impossible to keep any longer. We told the coach enough in the hope that he would help. That proved to be wishful thinking. He had no solutions and offered no empathy. Heidi and I bore our secrets to him, and it was as if we said nothing at all. We never heard from the coach again. Tennis and Millsaps had felt like a lifeline for Henry, and it disappeared in an instant.

Looking back, it was clear that the school and the coach had been conspiring. The next day we received a call from the school—a very formal, mostly one-sided conversation, as if scripted by attorneys. We were told that Henry had violated numerous school policies and needed to withdraw immediately. Heidi and I were asked to come to Jackson to pack him up and take him home.

We were devastated. All we wanted for Henry was a good college experience like what we had enjoyed. Like all his friends had enjoyed. That phone call dashed those hopes. We were getting ready to get in the car to go to Jackson when we got another call from the school saying Henry had been taken to a psychiatric hospital in Jackson. There had been an incident where Henry was standing in the middle of the road throwing food at cars. In my imagination I pictured an unkempt, bearded man, barefoot, dressed in sweats and hoodie, ranting and raving at passing cars. The kind of person we have all seen and done our best to avoid. You cannot imagine news like this. There's the self-pity that this is your life mixed with the anguish of watching your son circle the drain. Henry had been successful at Millsaps. He did well in school and was a beloved member of his tennis team. To watch his fall from grace was devastating. One of the problems with mental illness, as opposed to most other kinds of illnesses, is the lack of empathy for those suffering from it. I can understand why people hesitate to deal with someone in a state of psychosis. While they're in this state, they are difficult to be around—and may even seem dangerous. But it is important to understand that while they are in a state of psychosis, they are not psychotic. It is not *who* they are. It is a symptom of their disease. They are the same people you have always known and loved. But they live with the symptoms of their disease. Henry was a great kid suffering from a horrible illness. To judge him any other way was cruel. Though I was never concerned for my safety with Henry while he was in a state of psychosis, I can understand why others could be. Henry needed to be hospitalized during these episodes. With proper care, they end. Yet, when Henry recovered and reverted to his old self, some still treated him like a leper. Seeing his friends abandon him was hard on us and especially hard on Henry, who collected friends like people collect prized baseball cards. And then he lost them all.

Heidi and I drove to Jackson enveloped in sadness. We were hoping that the school would now admit that Henry was sick and not simply a discipline problem. We argued that he should be allowed to have some time off to get his disease under control. The school refused. They did not want him back. I am not sure why they took this approach. It made me question the notion and ideals of higher education and brought me right back to what had happened to Henry at Lawrenceville. No second chance. And ten years later it was more of the same. Exactly what lesson were they sending to Henry? You are a problem, but just not ours! Good luck and good riddance? We were yet again forced to help Henry navigate an educational system that was indifferent to him. Worse than indifferent, like dirt on their hands, they just wanted to wash it all away.

Heidi and I were back in a hospital dealing with a sick child with a disease few understood. We went to Henry's dorm to pack up his stuff. Up and down the stairs of his dorm, trip after trip, putting Henry's stuff in our car. Only eighteen months earlier we had made the same trip, but up those same stairs, and so full of joy and armed with a hope that had vanished overnight.

As we went up and down the stairs, we watched the kids pass by, doing their best to avoid us. In each kid we could see a life Henry would never have. None of them would make eye contact. Packing up Henry's places was always hard. This one was particularly brutal. No one came to help. Not a single friend, nor any coach. We were on an island that no one wanted to visit. It was a lonely place. Having a friend or coach stop by might have eased our pain. It might have eased our isolation. Our son was in a mental hospital. Life sucked, and no one seemed to care. If Henry were withdrawing from school to fight cancer, we would have been supported by an army of people. It wouldn't have been so damn lonely. We were in the fight of our lives. Alone.

chapter 20

MARDI GRAS

It was a grey day in February, cold and gloomy. Heidi and I were in the hospital in Jackson. We were beginning to see a pattern with Henry's episodes: they often seemed to happen after the holidays. Or maybe we just felt them more acutely during that time of the year. Our friends were all enjoying festive days with their families, while we were visiting our son in various psych wards. And this February, it was the week before Mardi Gras.

When I was young, we always went away for Mardi Gras. Most of the social clubs excluded Jews and Blacks, and my dad wanted nothing to do with it. As I got older, I sided with my dad. Every Mardi Gras since our own kids were little, we would go skiing at Copper Mountain. Finally, after years of not participating in any of the festivities, a friend asked if I wanted to ride in his place in Hermes. Hermes was the parade on the Friday night before the Tuesday of Mardi Gras. Hermes, it turns out, had always allowed Jews. That Friday was an all-day affair, starting with a lunch in the French Quarter and followed by a walking parade through the throngs filling the Quarter. It was a pleasant, sunny day as we walked behind the famous high school band, The St. Augustine Marching 100. We then headed to the Hilton hotel where we changed into our assigned costume. We were bussed with police escort uptown to the beginning of the parade route, where we boarded our floats. Hermes began at 5:30 p.m. The crowds were a sea of humanity, a flood of faces all screaming at me to throw them something. We rode for about two hours, and by the end I was spent. While the day had been long, it opened my eyes to the possibilities. So, when my friend asked me to join Hermes, I did. After a few years, one of my high school friends got a group of us together on the same float. Six idiots being towed through the streets of Uptown New Orleans to relive their glory days before thousands of people. We were always a little overserved or overbaked depending on the person, and we always had a great Friday night. As I sat in the hospital that Thursday night, I knew Hermes would not be in my weekend plans.

Heidi and I had planned our annual ski trip to Colorado, which was now in jeopardy as well. This was Henry's fourth hospitalization, and with each one we felt a new sense of urgency to find a treatment plan that worked. We found a well-regarded clinic in Arizona that was willing to take him so long as we could pay the $30,000 a month price tag. No insurance was willing to pay for places like these. Henry agreed to go. He would have said anything to get out of that psych ward in Jackson. Heidi and I planned to take him to Arizona, drop him off, and head to Copper Mountain for a few days of skiing.

I am well aware that our ability to pay for these treatment centers is a luxury few others have. Heidi and I were fortunate to have the money to help us navigate the hospitals and treatment centers. It is heartbreaking that, as a society, we leave those less fortunate to fend for themselves. Having gone through this process with money, it seems deeply unfair to those without. Yet another example of the dog-eat-dog world in which we live. And even though we had the money to get Henry into the best places, we were still losing our battle. Heidi and I learned the hard way that when it comes to bipolar disorder, no amount of money can fix the problem.

Our plan was to fly to Jackson to get Henry, then fly with him to Arizona. Henry had other ideas. He wanted to go home. We spent over two hours in a near empty Jackson airport begging him to go to the treatment center in Arizona. He refused, stating repeatedly that there was nothing wrong with him and that we were the ones with a problem. We were the ones using The System to keep him under our thumbs. After a high-pitched two hours of this back and forth, to our dismay, Henry called a taxi to take him to his car still in Jackson and took off. And in doing so, he destroyed all of our plans. For him. And for us. Heidi was a wreck, and I was emotionally exhausted. She and I spent the next thirty minutes fighting over what to do. Heidi wanted to go back to New Orleans, so she could keep an eye on Henry. I, being the selfish man that I am, wanted to go skiing. I know this makes me look bad. I had a son with a serious illness, loose and alone in New Orleans over Mardi Gras no less, and I wanted to ski. It wasn't that I didn't care about him or love him. I knew Henry needed help.

But I needed a break. It was like I had just run three marathons, and now, they were asking me to run one more. I had reached terminal velocity. Like an overheated engine, I was about to burn out. In my view, a little time skiing was all I needed to recharge. And I knew Heidi needed it, too. Finally, in that sad and empty Jackson airport, she agreed.

It was getting late and arranging the flight to Colorado was difficult. It involved an overnight stay in Houston. When we finally arrived at the mountain the next day, we called Kate, who said Henry was home and doing fine. Once again, Kate to the rescue. I hated relying on my youngest daughter, but in my overwhelmed and vulnerable state, unable to find a way to fix Henry's problem, almost unable to go on, that is exactly what I did. I let go of some of the control I held onto so tightly, and Heidi and I managed to relax a little and had a good trip.

chapter 21

WEEKEND IN JAIL

When we returned to New Orleans, Henry returned to living with us at home, and no one was happy about it. You would think that after all his hospitalizations and all the chaos, he would be ready to accept he had a problem. You would be wrong. I believe he knew that there was something off. He just didn't know what it was.

Heidi, having read volumes on the disease, understood this better than me. I viewed his lack of awareness as a sign of weakness. I was wrong. No one wants to be sick. No one asks to have cancer. Henry did not want to have bipolar disorder. It was his biology playing a cruel trick on him, and he was powerless to stop it. How scary it must be to go from being in charge to being unable to control your thoughts. Yet somehow, at times, I found myself struggling to maintain my empathy for his condition. I left him alone on the battlefield. Henry fought it with the only weapons he felt he had. His first line of defense had been to become vegan. At the time I thought he was being compulsive. I now see he was trying to regain control over his life and was using his diet as a defense against this thing he could not understand.

His second line of defense was to move out of our house.

Henry wanted to go back to Jackson. He wanted to rent an apartment and find work. Much to our surprise, he got a job teaching tennis at a public school near Millsaps in Jackson. Once again, instead of insisting he get help as a precondition to our continued support, we were all too happy to find him an apartment in Jackson and get him settled in. We were as bad as Henry in our inability to accept our new reality. We were desperate for him to be "normal."

Heidi embraced the diagnosis of bipolar disorder. She read everything she could about mental illness and the stories of those who had gone through similar ordeals. Not me. I thought I knew everything, and I was convinced that the stories of others would be of no use. My failure to accept my new reality didn't help me, Henry, or my family. On the contrary, it rendered me unable to handle the problem at all. He had just had a momentous year at Millsaps without any medication, and I was confused. I clung to the hope that this was just a phase he would outgrow. Under the pressure of having a child who was mentally ill, I was unable to become the person I needed to be.

If I could go back in time, I would seek out the help Heidi was searching for. Yet again, she was trying to show me the way, and, yet again, I ignored her. My ego was being tested, and I was failing miserably. Heidi was looking for help, but all she got from me was attitude.

Henry moved back to Jackson. We could track his car and see where he went. He had no idea. With this insight into his daily movement, his gambling issues had really come to the forefront. Poker was his game, and he was good at it. While he won often, when he lost, he lost spectacularly. Similar to his tennis game, he was incredibly aggressive in poker. It often served him well. Until it didn't. He read everything he could about poker and played every day. The closest place to play in Jackson was Vicksburg, about forty-five minutes due west on the banks of the Mississippi, and I could see his car in the parking lot on most days. He would take his paycheck from his coaching job and use it to fund his poker. Soon, he had $10,000 in savings. He didn't want me to see his winnings, so he opened an account at a different bank to which I had no access. He never asked us for money, so I assumed the good hands kept coming.

I do know that Henry loved working with the kids on his team. He had always had an affinity for kids. And kids loved him back. He never felt judged by them. He worked with children under twelve, and they hadn't yet learned the art of shaming. They accepted him for who he was. He didn't need to live up to some expectation of what he should be. To those kids he was just Henry. That fun and funny guy who was great at tennis. He was one of them.

While Henry seemed to be thriving in Jackson, he remained obsessed with Millsaps. He would hang around on the outskirts of campus, hoping to run into some of his old teammates. The school got wind of this and warned Heidi and me that he needed to stay away. They treated Henry like he was "a danger to their community." But was he really? Institutions often jump to the worst possible scenarios and leave compassion at home. There was no middle ground for them—yet the middle ground is where learning takes place. And while Heidi and I believed that Henry was being unfairly singled out, we still had to warn him to stay away. Heidi and I could give him no good reason for this rule because we saw no good reason.

Henry lived close to both campus and his job. He used a Onewheel to commute. Imagine a skateboard with an electric wheel in the center. He would ride to the courts where he coached his young team. On this particular Friday, on his ride home, Henry stopped to watch a softball game. Someone hit a homerun that went over the fence. He retrieved the ball and threw it back. At this point someone in an unmarked car yelled out his name and told him not to move. He got scared and ran. The next thing he knew, two police cars cornered him and arrested him for resisting arrest. The person who had yelled at him was an off-duty police officer working for the school. Apparently, Henry was a wanted man, having risen to the status of a "dangerous" person at Millsaps. All he had done was throw a softball back over a fence, yet that had been enough to warrant a high-end confrontation, with the off-duty officer calling for backup. Some people can't believe things like this actually happen. That the police would ever do that. But it did, and they do.

The police made him leave his Onewheel on the side of the road. They handcuffed him, took him to jail, and booked him for resisting arrest. It was a Friday afternoon, and he was stuck there until a bail hearing could be had on Monday morning. My son, who had thrown a ball over a fence, was forced to spend the weekend in jail in Jackson. This was Henry's first time dealing with the criminal justice system, and it would not be his last. And while we could have afforded bail, the system was in no hurry to grant it. As much as we tried to avoid a weekend in jail, there appeared to be little we could do. It's not a line in a country song, but it should be: "Don't get arrested in Jackson on a Friday night." For Henry, all he saw was a system set up to keep him down. It was the police who took him to the psych wards. It was the police who snatched him off that Onewheel in Jackson. And thus began in Henry a profound distrust of the police. His father was beginning to feel the same way.

First thing Monday morning, my brother was able to get Henry released without bail. Of course, his Onewheel was long gone. Henry had missed his team's tennis match on Saturday because of his weekend "retreat," so the school informed him that they "had to let him go." Henry had been fired, and it broke his heart. He loved those kids. He left Jackson a broken man and a lost boy. He returned to New Orleans defeated.

I had an important meeting I could not miss, so I asked Kate to go with Heidi to Jackson to pack up Henry's apartment. I felt bad for Kate. Having returned to New Orleans after college to begin working with Heidi, Henry's energy twin was getting sucked into the drama. This disease takes its toll on the siblings. But while Patti, who had first moved to New York to start her career then to Chicago, was not around for most of this, Kate had a front row seat. We relied on Kate in unhealthy ways. The boundaries grew very blurred, and we often drove through them like a Panzer tank over a wooden fence. In looking back, this is a profound regret. When you're in the middle of the chaos, any help is welcome. So, we leaned on Kate hard, and she never let us down. She never complained. Off she went with Heidi to Jackson to help pack up Henry's apartment. Kate was devastated by the experience. Of course she was. Seeing the state in which Henry lived was a shock. She was upset for days. While we would have to pack Henry up at least one more time, we never put Kate in that situation again.

chapter 22

CROSS-COUNTRY TRIP

Henry was home again. His only source of income was delivering food and working a little at A's and Aces. And there was poker. The dreaded poker. Henry would enter tournaments where the top prize was as much as $20,000. He won $7,500 at one of these. The cycle was always the same. He would deliver food until he had enough to play poker. He would win, build up a nest egg, then lose it playing fast and loose. Rinse, repeat. The cycle went on for a long time. He never asked us for money. I was proud of the fact that he was so good at poker. I was searching for the silver linings in Henry's life, and poker was all I could find. I should have been proud of the fact that he was in the fight of his life and seemed to be doing the best he could. I should have been proud of how hard he was fighting for any semblance of normal. But we Friedlers need markers for our success, and poker was all I had. Poker gave us something to talk about, a connection other than his disease. He would light up when he talked about poker, so we shared stories of hands won and lost. At this point it was the only intimacy Henry allowed me.

But poker can only go so far, and I could see Henry slipping away. I could tell he was restless as his anger grew. Henry had long been skeptical of all authority. Who could blame him? He had been on the wrong end too many times. Everywhere he went, the system had betrayed him. In his endless search for somewhere else, America had become the evil empire. He wanted out. Like in preschool, Henry became fixated on a map. Henry and his maps. This time, instead of Africa, it was Germany. For the past few years, he had romanticized the idea of life in Germany. In his mind Germany was where he would be healthy and happy. Having fallen down some rabbit hole on the internet touting the beauty of life in Germany, he told us repeatedly that college and health care were free there. He knew that college and his hospitalizations had been expensive for us, and he hated the fact that he was beholden to us, even though we never held that over him. Henry was desperate to regain a measure of control, and he wanted his freedom, both financially and emotionally.

About a month after we had moved him back home from Jackson, I was at the office getting ready to leave for the day. I had a tennis match scheduled for five and was clearing out my emails when Heidi called. "Tripp, I was passing in front of the computer upstairs and saw a boarding pass for Henry to Germany," she said frantically. "There are three boarding passes, one from New Orleans to New York, one from New York to Iceland, then one from Iceland to Germany. The first flight leaves in thirty minutes."

It took me a few seconds to process this new insanity. "I don't understand. Henry bought a ticket to Germany, and he leaves in thirty minutes?"

"Exactly," she shouted. "We need to do something. If he gets to Germany, we'll lose him forever!"

I fired questions at Heidi, knowing she had no answers. "How did he buy the tickets? What card did he use? When did he buy it? Can you see it on the screen? What airline?"

Heidi was able to find that he had bought a ticket that day on JetBlue to NYC, then a flight on Ryanair from NYC to Germany, all using a card in my name. I looked at the JetBlue flight and saw it was delayed an hour. A drop of good luck in an ocean of shit. I called JetBlue and informed them that my son had taken my card and bought the flight without my permission. That he had bipolar disorder, was not well, and could not be allowed to board the flight. They assured me that they would cancel the ticket and that he would not be allowed on the plane. I called Ryanair next. They were not so helpful and refused to cancel the ticket. But I had stopped Henry from getting to NYC, so getting a refund from the assholes at Ryanair was low on my list of priorities.

I then called Henry, dreading what was sure to be an explosive response. "Henry," I said in the calmest voice I could muster at the time, "I know you are at the airport. I know you bought a ticket to Germany. I canceled it, and you are not going to be allowed on the plane."

"You can't do that," he said. "That card is in my name. It's my card."

That was technically true, as it was his name on the card. But it was our card. We paid for it; it was based on our credit.

He knew that and didn't fight me hard. But he was pissed. He understood that Germany was not happening.

"How did you even know what I was doing?" he asked in a surprisingly calm voice.

"You left the boarding pass on the computer, and Mom saw it." I replied. "What were you thinking? Did you even have a plan?" My voice was getting edgier. I knew I should have tried to stay calm, that I should have deescalated the situation, yet I felt my face getting hotter. My voice grew louder, and I could feel everyone's temperature rising a notch. Henry fed off my tone.

"I'm a grown ass man and can do whatever I want." He was mad, mostly at his stupidity for leaving the boarding pass on the screen.

"Henry, I am in no mood to argue," I said trying to regain my composure. "Please come home, and we can talk about it. You are not getting on that flight. I can have the police take you out of the airport, or you can leave on your own. Either way you need to come home."

"Okay, I'll leave. You're an asshole! Can't you just let me live my life!" he shouted before hanging up on me.

Crisis averted. Heidi was happy I had handled it but was not looking forward to Hurricane Henry coming back uptown for a direct hit. Neither of us were, but it was better than the alternative. Now that we could breathe, I began to contemplate the lunacy of what had just happened. What if Heidi had not been near the computer? We would have had no idea where he was. I could have tracked the car and seen it was at the airport, but beyond that we'd have no clue. He had bought a one-way ticket to Germany and driven his car to the airport. Had he planned to keep it there for a few years? Didn't seem that he'd given this plan too much thought. Yet another example of manic behavior. At least he was not yet in psychosis.

I checked the car to make sure he was on his way home. Henry's Pilot was moving but instead of heading east toward our home, it was going west. Maybe the GPS was acting up. I told Heidi, and we started watching my phone screen like it was our favorite TV show. It soon became clear that he was on the interstate heading away from New Orleans. As we did not want him to know we could track his car, we were in a quandary. I called him to ask if he was on his way home. He said yes, clearly a lie. Two hours later he was near Lake Charles, Louisiana, not far from the Texas border. We called him again. This time he said he was not coming home, that he had decided to drive out west.

Henry was sucking all of the oxygen out of our lives. It's terribly hard to watch your kids struggle. Some struggles are simpler because they feel unavoidable or one-sided. Being broken up with. Not getting that role in the school play. A friend who disappears into a new interest. Henry's was not simple. A sickness that hides in you and interrupts your most fundamental relationships, your most basic ambitions for any institutional belonging, is not one-sided, it's endlessly petrifying. While grateful he was not on an airplane to Germany, we were concerned as to where he was going now. We had a sick child who was heading west in a car, destination unknown. Our fears of his disappearance overseas had not been assuaged; they had morphed into a panic of when and where he was going to stop. It didn't really help to constantly refresh our screen. The miles went by in hours, not seconds. At first, we would check every ten minutes. When it was clear which direction he was heading, we switched to every hour. At this point he was nearing Houston and then went past it. We were tired and needed to get some sleep. I had never needed anything stronger than marijuana to calm my nerves, but this was different. I was prescribed Klonopin to help when the anxiety overwhelmed me. Tonight was one of those nights. When I woke up the next morning, he was in west Texas, on his way to New Mexico.

We were now playing a real-life version of Where's Waldo. My first hunch was Vegas. He loved poker, and, depending on how flush he was, I thought he might head there to test his mettle. I kept trying to figure out what route he would take. Heidi was profoundly worried. She let all her darkest thoughts swirl around in her brain like a dancing devil. I tend to be more optimistic than she is, though at this point my devil was starting to dance, too. I had my own business, a wife, two other kids, yet I spent the entirety of my day on MapQuest. My loss of control infuriated me. My son was sick, he was on the road, and there was absolutely nothing I could do about it.

When he passed his exit to Vegas, I was back to square one. At this point there was only one place he could head to, the city of Angels. At least there, I had one more trick up my sleeve.

chapter 23

STEPHEN

Stephen Godchaux is one of my oldest friends. His uncle and my dad were business partners. Stephen was a year ahead of me at Newman, and, although we grew up together, by the time he was in seventh grade, he was way too cool to hang with sixth graders like me. He was, and still is, very athletic and extremely attractive. Stephen never had any issues with sports or girls, though I believe he was better at girls than sports. My mom was a huge fan of Stephen, especially after he had been accepted to Dartmouth. My SAT scores were horrible, and mom figured that Stephen, being the genius she thought him to be, could tutor me for the SATs.

She paid Stephen to tutor me. This is what tutoring meant: we drove up to The Butterfly, a pretty and popular spot in Audubon Park on the banks of the Mississippi river, parked, and smoked copious amounts of marijuana. As Stephen was the one getting paid, he supplied the pot. I don't believe the SAT test ever came up. Neither did my scores. Fortunately, I was good at tennis, and Amherst found a spot for me.

Stephen took a year off after college, and we ended up in the same class at Tulane Law School. Now that we were classmates, we started hanging out together. We each had our own little cliques, but we would see each other quite often and share notes on the cute girls we were dating. And this is where the story gets even weirder. By our senior year, Stephen was telling me about this cute girl who worked in the bookstore, Heidi Hackley, the future Mrs. Heidi Hackley Friedler. Stephen met my wife before I did. They dated briefly but were such good friends they became roommates instead. So not only was Stephen one of my closest friends, he and Heidi were close as well.

Stephen graduated and then went to work in San Francisco for a big firm. Like me, he also decided law was not for him. He applied and was accepted to The Yale School of Drama as a playwright. Stephen went on to write for such shows as *Roseanne*, *Spin City*, and *Dead Like Me*, just to name a few. He had been living in Santa Monica for the past twenty years, and he visited Heidi and me often in New Orleans. He was our only friend who had a key to our house.

Stephen never married nor had any kids of his own, so he was always very close to all of my kids. He even used the name Henry Friedler as a character in one of his TV pilots which was filmed in New Orleans. When I realized that Henry might be on his way to Los Angeles, I called Stephen and hatched a plan. I knew that if I called Henry and suggested that he do anything, I would be shot down like a duck over southwest Louisiana: quickly and violently. Stephen, on the other hand, was someone Henry thought was cool. If Stephen called Henry to catch up and could get him to say he was on the road and on the way to L.A., then Stephen could invite him to stay with him in Santa Monica. Stephen was all in, and the plan worked like a charm. I think Henry was subconsciously heading to L.A. because of Stephen. And just like that I was back in control.

Henry arrived in Los Angeles a few days later and drove to Stephen's. He was tired from his ride and went to sleep. Stephen called to say he was there and safe. As an accomplice, he did a great job of keeping Heidi and me informed. Unfortunately, because Stephen cares so much about our family, he soon became consumed by Henry's every waking moment. Every time Henry left the house for more than a few hours, my phone would ring. Stephen wanted me to track Henry. On one such day, I told Stephen that Henry was in Commerce, California. Stephen said that's where the poker rooms near L.A. were. Of course they were. About a week into this, Stephen called with some anxiety in his voice: "He wants to go to San Francisco. That's a terrible idea." No shit. Stephen was soon to find out he had no control over Henry, either. In a slight role reversal, I had to tutor in The Art of Henry. I assured Stephen that Henry would return. I told him that Henry was still manic and was probably just getting restless. Henry was gone no more than two days before calling Stephen and asking if he could come back. Stephen welcomed Henry back enthusiastically, of course. Henry stayed another five days. Stephen and I agreed that his mania was ending. Henry finally called me and asked if he could come home. I said, of course, his mother and I would love for him to come home. I think Stephen aged ten years in three weeks. And I'm confident he was happy that he had stayed childless. Stephen gave Henry a few hundred dollars and saw him off.

chapter 24

"Dad, where's the insurance information for the car?" Henry asked when I answered his call the next day. Never a great opening line in a conversation with your kid.

"It's in the glove compartment. Is everything okay, Henry?"

"I'm about two hours outside of L.A. and had to take a dump super bad, so I got off the highway and ran a stop sign to get to this gas station," he answered. "This cop pulled me over." Then I heard Henry talking to the cop. "I have to go so bad! Please let me go." Henry hung up on me.

I didn't hear anything for a good hour. Henry wouldn't answer his phone. My anxiety was now at DEFCON 5. An hour later I got a call from a number I did not recognize. It was Henry. He was in jail. Clearly things had escalated.

"Dad, this is bullshit," he said, "I was in the car and told the cop I had to go to the bathroom really bad. He said too bad and stay in the car. I told him again how bad I had to go, and he told me again to stay in the car or get 'kicked to the curb.'"

In his panicked state, Henry thought the cop was telling him he could get out and sit on the curb. As he started getting out of the car, the cop went berserk and tried to grab Henry. Henry, with his well-earned distrust of police, took off. He ran around the block and got back in his car. The next thing he knew there were four police cars. They broke the passenger side window, pulled him out of the car, and then arrested him for felony resisting arrest.

This seemed like Jackson all over again. Felony resisting arrest did not seem like Henry. I suspected an overly aggressive officer.

"Dad. This is a serious jail," he said in a concerned voice. "They have some pretty bad people in here. Please help. I didn't do anything wrong." I could hear the terror in his voice.

"Henry, I'll try to help. Is there anyone there I can talk to?"

He handed the phone to an officer nearby. The officer explained that Henry had been arrested for felony resisting arrest, a much more serious charge than merely resisting arrest. If I wanted him released, I would need to post bail. Then, he gave me the number of a bail bondsman. Heidi frantically Googled Banning, California. It's about one hundred miles east of L.A, twenty-five miles west of Palm Springs, and in the center of nowhere.

For those who have never had the joy of a brush with the criminal justice system, I can best describe it in two words: *fucked up*. The whole structure is set up to squeeze as much money out of you as possible. The first step is the bail bondsman. I am confident the officer who referred me got a commission. I called the bondsman and was told that since it was a *felony* resisting arrest that the bond would be $10,000, and I had to pay a 10% nonrefundable fee of $1,000. It was now midnight in New Orleans, and I had to fax him our credit information as well as a host of other information. An hour later our credit was approved, the bond issued, and Henry was released. It was five in the morning in Banning when Henry walked out of jail. It was another Klonopin night for me and probably a sleepless one for Heidi.

After dealing with the bail, we now had to get Henry back to his car. This was a $20 cab ride to the tow yard. The towing company, yet another willing player in this system, charged $250 for the towing fee. To get Henry back on the road set me back about $1,300. I could afford it. The ones least likely to afford it are the ones most likely to get caught up in the system. They either sit in jail, lose their car, or both. Quite the little scam.

Henry finished the drive back to New Orleans with his passenger side window taped over. He now had to fight the felony charge. I knew he needed a lawyer who was local, so I called Stephen. Stephen called his agent, who knew the perfect guy. The typical Hollywood fixer. That guy set us back $10,000. He told me that once he requested the video from the police cams this would go away or at least be knocked down to a misdemeanor. This was not his first rodeo. Before any of that could happen, we would need to get a court date, and Henry would have to appear in person, to plead not guilty.

I had meetings in New Orleans, so Heidi took Henry back to California for his hearing. Once again, I somehow let Heidi do the heavy lifting. Their court time was 9 a.m. the next day, so they rented a car at LAX for the drive to Banning and spent the night in Palm Springs. The next morning Heidi and Henry got to court a few minutes early, meeting their lawyers for the first time on the courthouse steps. They were in and out like a fast-food joint and back at the airport for their 1 p.m. flight back to New Orleans. Henry would have everything expunged from his record if he stayed out of trouble in California for a year. Not a problem. California would not be on Henry's itinerary for a while. I kept thinking about those people who could not afford the solutions I could afford. What do they do? They spend time in jail. They have a felony on their record. They lose their job, their car, and have a tough time getting a new one of either. Seems like a terrible cycle of injustice, and all because you can't afford to play in the system.

For now, we put it all in our rearview mirror and moved on. In the middle of all this turmoil, Henry enrolled at the University of New Orleans. He was about two semesters short of graduating from college, and all of us wanted that to happen. He was back to living at home, delivering food, and coaching kids at A's and Aces. He was also playing poker and winning, so he was flush with cash.

During this relative period of calm, Heidi was away at girls' weekend in Boston. Kate and I were having dinner.

"You know mom was at Britt and Nan's house, and she loved their dog," she said.

I looked up with great interest.

"What kind of dog is it?" I asked, much too quickly.

"A Lagotto Romagnolo."

"A what? What kind of dog is that? How big?"

"They are about thirty pounds and are hypoallergenic," she replied. "Their dog's name is Mia, and mom loved her."

I had always been a dog person. When Heidi and I were first married, I had two Chesapeake Bay retrievers, Humboldt and Nikki. Humboldt eventually got old and blind, and we had to put him down at age twelve. After Kate was born, Heidi could not handle three kids and a dog, so we gave Nikki to a loving home on a farm in Mississippi. Since then, Heidi had vetoed dogs in the house. And I had to agree that raising three kids was hard enough. Time moved on, and we remained dogless.

"She made me promise not to tell you," Kate said with a big grin. "She knew you had no patience and would want one right away."

Four weeks later we had Bella, a beautiful white Lagotto. Heidi fell in love with Bella, as did I, as did Kate and Patti, and as did Henry.

Henry started the fall semester at UNO and seemed eager to move forward. Once again, we were lulled into a sense that maybe this had all been a nightmare that was soon ending. That Henry was "growing out of it." Kate was working for Heidi and doing well. She had saved some money and was looking for a place to live. Heidi and I wanted to find a double where Kate could live on one side and Henry the other. Again, we were leaning on Kate in very unhealthy ways. And again, Kate was agreeing to be leaned upon. We found the perfect place about two miles from us in a cute Uptown neighborhood. It was a perfect place for Kate, with a small apartment attached for Henry. Both he and Kate were excited and moved in around September. You're only as happy as your least happy child, and, in this rare moment, all three seemed happy. During these increasingly rare moments, Heidi and I used to joke by putting our fingers in the shape of a hashtag and saying, "Hashtag blessed." The phrase originated on Instagram, and, while it started for us as tongue and cheek, it became shorthand for happiness. I even got a hashtag tattooed on the inside of my wrist to remind me of times like these.

Henry was trying to live a more wholesome life. He had to know something was off, yet he appeared unwilling to accept it could be a disease. His ego couldn't take that he was different from everyone else. From all his friends. So, he did what he could within his own powers. Henry quit doing drugs of any kind, including marijuana. Committed to living a clean, vegan life, he even went so far as to refuse to wear any clothes made from animal products. Like everything Henry did, he went all out.

Around this time, Henry began to feel that a capped tooth was also causing problems. When he was twelve, Heidi had gotten one of his teeth capped. For some unknown reason, Henry was now certain that the capped tooth was part of the problem. He wanted the cap removed. He had just won $5,000 in a poker tournament. Feeling emboldened, he went from dentist to dentist, and each one refused. There was nothing wrong with his cap. But Henry was persistent, a trait he probably picked up from me. He kept going until he found a willing dentist. We were clueless this was happening until one of the dentists called us. When we confronted Henry, he told us it was *his* mouth and *his* teeth, and he could do whatever he wanted. Henry was so handsome, and Heidi begged him not to do it. It was like talking to a wall. Two days later we saw the results. It was not pretty. Henry was already having a tough time in life and now, when he smiled, his left canine was just small and pointy. Luckily and sadly, Henry rarely smiled.

And then, out of nowhere, Henry told us that he was leaving the next day for Hawaii to live on a commune. He had already purchased the ticket, and, as his classes were all online, he could finish them from Hawaii. There was absolutely nothing we could do. I asked him where he was going, and he told me he was going to an eco-village called Cinderland on the Big Island. Their vision was a place where people lived in ecological harmony. They wanted a community that tried to use sustainable, responsible agriculture using natural methods. To live there you were required to pay a fee of three hundred dollars a month and to help maintain the community. Henry was excited and assured us that he would finish his semester and stay in touch with us. He said he would be picked up at the airport by the commune. We wanted to show our support, so we took him to the airport. And Heidi and I had our usual foolproof plan in place: fingers crossed and hoping for the best. So off he went, crooked smile and all.

chapter 25

PARADISE LOST

As we feared, Henry did not find nirvana in Hawaii. He was now five hours and five time zones behind us, but we were able to track his movements via his cell phone. Living on a remote part of the island, cell phone reception was iffy to nonexistent. He was essentially "off the grid." If he had a manic episode in Hawaii, there would be nothing we could do. Henry called infrequently, and, when he did, he needed something. He was still taking his courses and passing, but I don't know how.

Meanwhile, Heidi and I started going to Al Anon meetings, which were incredibly helpful. Al Anon was founded in 1951 to help families of those who have loved ones suffering from addiction. Even though Henry did not have a drug or alcohol problem, the effects on Heidi and me were similar. He was spiraling down the drain of life, and we could only watch. Coming to grips with our helplessness was the same for us as it was for parents of addicts. If someone had asked me at the time, I would have said that Henry had no power over his situation, whereas addicts could control their behavior. It seemed to me that addicts *chose* to be addicts. But with the help of Al Anon, I came to view this differently. No one with a mental illness chose their condition any more than someone with cancer or alcoholism chose theirs. I came to understand that addiction is a mental illness. It is not one anyone would choose. Addicts also suffer from public shaming. And perhaps worse, people believe, as I did, that the addict has a choice. Al Anon helped me see that none of our loved ones chose the path they were on. Al Anon preaches to let go, accept your reality, and come to peace with the fact that you have no control over the situation. Hearing all the sad stories in the room comforted me. Misery does love company. I began to think I could let go and let the chips fall where they may. I began to think I had this control thing beat. Then my cell phone rang.

"Dad, I'm running out of money, and I had to sell my phone," he said. "So don't try calling. I really don't know how much longer I can stay here. It's not what I thought it would be. It is very cliquey, and no one's talking to me. And these people who run the place want you to work but won't pay you. And then they charge you for everything."

My fixer mode went into high gear. "You need a cell phone, Henry. Go to the store and find a cheap phone, and I'll transfer money to your card. Do you want to come home? I'm happy to buy you a ticket."

"No. I want to try to make it here," he replied. "I think I can. Let me try a little longer. I'll get a new phone. Thanks for the help."

Did I just hear Henry say thanks? I had not heard that in an exceedingly long time. He must be in a pretty bad way. My mind started racing, and the images were not pretty. I knew he was not manic. It sounded more like he was down. Either way I had at least talked to him, and we hadn't had a fight. I was happy about that. And I had convinced him to go into town and get another phone. Happy about that, too. Silver linings.

Heidi and I were still worried but at least we had a connection to Henry if we needed one. We were feeling pretty bleak. Then, we received an invitation to a good friend's sixtieth birthday party. Hans is married to Kate, who I've known since freshman year of college. Kate, Hans, Heidi, and I have all been good friends for decades. And Hans and Kate were having a big birthday blowout near their home in the Berkshires. The party was going to be a real shin dig and one of the few bright spots in an otherwise dark existence. Hans has had a fascinating life in business and in philanthropy. Along the way he's collected a lot of interesting friends. Heidi and I were excited to spend a long weekend in the Berkshires with them. We just wanted to have some fun. It had been a while.

We flew into Albany, rented a car, and drove to Stockbridge for the Friday night welcome party at Kate and Hans' house. We knew a few people and met many more who we didn't. We left relatively early, so we could check into the hotel before it got too late. We unpacked our bags and went straight to bed, excited for the next day.

We woke up to a beautiful, sunny day. It was early December in Massachusetts and on the warm side. One of those perfect days in New England. The leaves had fallen off the trees, but the air was clear and crisp. The sun was doing its job so that forty-five degrees felt like sixty. It was the kind of day that makes you happy to be alive. There was nothing planned until 11 a.m., so we were able to lounge around in our room. It brought back memories of what life had been like before pandemonium encompassed our lives. I vividly remembered the feeling of those lazy weekends on vacations, just Heidi and me without a care in the world.

Our vacation routine was not complicated. Heidi loved to sleep in, so I would usually get up, exercise, and stretch. I would get a local newspaper and coffee for the two of us. I would lounge in the room, waiting for her to wake up. That feeling of leisure, that freedom from all worries had disappeared from our lives for a long time and had been replaced with constant anxiety and bickering about how to manage all of our worries. For a brief moment in time, I forgot them. And I think Heidi did, too. She was smiling like the young girl I met in 1985.

Thirty-three years later, we were enjoying a beautiful crisp day in New England and preparing for an even better night. The hotel was across the street from the venue, so we walked over at the appointed hour for cocktails. Heidi looked elegant in her cream-colored Chanel sweater dress, and we were both looking forward to the evening. I was enjoying a great conversation and deep into my second glass of red wine when my cell phone rang. It was Henry. Of course it was Henry.

I excused myself and found a more private space, so I could hear. He was upset and wanted to come home immediately. He let me know that his life in Hawaii had been hard.

It was not what he thought it would be. He insisted on leaving right away. I'm not sure what had happened, nor was I sure that I would ever know. All I did know was that now I had to get Henry a ticket, find a flight, and get him to the airport. So, I had to get to work in the middle of a terrific cocktail party that I really wanted to be a part of. I got my travel agent on the phone for a three-way call with Henry. Forty-five minutes later it seemed we had a plan that could work, but Henry had only an hour to get to the airport and that was pressing it. So, even though we had a solution, there was still stress on my end as to whether he would make the flight. I got back just as the cocktail party was wrapping up. The good news was that Heidi hadn't had to deal with this and had made a bunch of new friends. In the big scheme of things, what I had to deal with that evening was nothing, of course. Yet, I still felt cheated. It seemed no matter where I went, Henry followed me. About forty-five minutes later, he texted saying all was good, he had made his flight, and he would be home late Sunday night. We would be back home as well, so we could pick him up at the airport. I downed another drink, maybe two, and did my best to enjoy the night. I was in good spirits. Henry was coming home. He was safe and returning in one piece. Plus, Chrissy Hyde and the Pretenders were the evening entertainment, so things could be a lot worse. We danced and had a great night. Tomorrow would come soon enough.

When Henry returned, he moved into the apartment next to Kate. He liked having his own place, and we liked him not living with us, though it did make it difficult to keep an eye on him. At least Kate was next door. As usual, she sacrificed some of her time to check on Henry. It was mid-December, and we had planned a small family Christmas. About a week before Christmas, Henry started to appear more disheveled. He quit showering and wore the same clothes for days on end. We all felt another round of mania was around the corner. The holiday season was upon us, and we were in a quandary. We knew he was deteriorating. At this point, we also knew his diagnosis was clearly bipolar disorder. After three years and five hospital stays, I accepted the obvious. At least my enemy had a name.

As often happened, Henry's mania morphed into psychosis, making it clear that we would need to hospitalize him again. Not the Christmas we had wanted. So, once again I drove over to the coroner's office to get my 72-hour hold. I was becoming an expert at that—not the sort of thing one wants to get good at. Heidi and I dreaded having to use it, as Henry would never forgive us. It was looking to be a bad few days.

No matter how many times we had seen Henry become psychotic, each new episode was scary. This time was no different, and I was about to call the police when Kate called.

"Dad, the police are here," she said trying not to cry. "You need to come now. Henry sprayed an anarchy symbol on his car in red paint, and one of the neighbors called the police. They didn't know it was his car and were concerned. He also was spraying the front porch when the police showed up. They have him in the back of the police car. I don't know what to do."

It is crazy to say, but I was relieved. Now, I didn't have to make the call to have him picked up. I drove over to their house where the police were waiting. I told them he had bipolar disorder and showed them my 72-hour hold. I also explained that the car Henry defaced was his car. They were extremely nice and instead of taking Henry to jail, they took him to the hospital. It was December 24th. Merry Christmas, everyone.

chapter 26

WORST CHRISTMAS EVER

Christmas in a mental ward is no Norman Rockwell painting. And hospitals are short staffed over the holidays. It seems doctors and nurses want to take off for vacation as well. When we went to visit Henry on Christmas Day, it was even more depressing than usual. No one really wants to be there on Christmas, and the lack of effort was impressive. Everything was a little harder and everyone a little less friendly. As usual, we went through security before we were allowed in. No one was especially helpful at security, but that day was unusually hard. The guard was curt with us. As if he had a better place to be and as if being there at all was all our fault. Henry was no happier to see us. "I can't believe you did it again. You put me in here. You are evil."

"Henry, your neighbor called the police," I replied. "We didn't. You were spray painting cars, and they didn't know who you were. This one is not on us."

"Well, you could have kept me out," he hissed back. "You came over and talked to the police. You could have gotten me released."

He was not wrong. Yet, there was no way we were going to allow him to keep going on the path he was on. Henry needed the help that he could only get in a hospital. This was a short visit, that Christmas Day. Henry wanted nothing to do with us and told us not to come back.

We did catch one break. Henry was placed in the Tulane wing of the University Medical Center under the care of Dr. Ashley Weiss. Dr. Weiss was a D.O, Doctor of Osteopathic Medicine. D.O.s are trained to look beyond a patient's symptoms to understand how lifestyle and environmental factors impact a patient's well-being. They are trained to treat the whole person. In addition, Dr. Weiss developed and founded the Early Psychosis Intervention Clinic (EPIC-NOLA) in 2015. EPIC is affiliated with Tulane and focuses on providing comprehensive care for adolescents and young adults experiencing their first episode of psychosis associated with the emergence of severe mental illness, such as bipolar disorder and diseases on the schizophrenia-spectrum. She was the perfect doctor for Henry. But because it was Christmas week, Henry would not see her until after January 1. Before that he saw a series of interns who seemed young enough to be my children. There was no continuity of care. Henry was hospitalized until January 4.

It was during this stay that one of the doctors diagnosed Henry as having schizophrenia. This diagnosis really got our attention and upset Heidi even more than she already was. It is interesting in the world of mental health how different diagnoses carry different connotations. For some reason we were okay with him having bipolar disorder. There were plenty of stories about people who have gone on to lead productive lives having bipolar disorder. We had never heard any such stories about schizophrenia. In fact, we had never heard one such story. The diagnosis of schizophrenia terrified us. Those were the people who hear voices. But Henry had never heard voices.

We refused to accept the schizophrenia diagnosis. What we would later learn about mental illness is that it is one big spectrum. A range of colors on a terrifying rainbow. And when we were finally able to speak with Dr. Weiss, she didn't believe that Henry had schizophrenia either. She felt comfortable that he had bipolar disorder with psychotic features. What a relief that he only had bipolar disorder with psychotic features.

EPIC-NOLA had an outpatient program for Henry, and they also offered counseling for parents. And this is where Serena dropped into our lives like an angel from heaven. We had been doing this all alone for many years now, and, while we had Andre, this was not his area of expertise. Serena, on the other hand, only dealt with patients or parents of patients who had either bipolar disorder or schizophrenia. Serena was the one who got us to understand that the diagnosis didn't matter as much as making sure that Henry improved. Meeting with Serena once a week helped Heidi and me. And she was instrumental in getting Henry to participate in their program. We felt for the first time in our long odyssey that we had an ally with expert knowledge. We had found our community.

Henry was less excited. He was still taking the position that he was fine and didn't need any help. The only reason he went was to keep us off his back and to get out of the hospital. He felt it was a total waste of time.

We planned a ski trip for my birthday. We felt there was a good team in place, and we could safely leave New Orleans. We were wrong. We had been in Colorado for two days when Nigel, my next-door neighbor, texted me a disturbing picture. It was a photo of Henry's car taken from the rear. He had decided to ram our garage door instead of opening it. The car was in the garage with a crumpled door on top of it. The back of his Honda was open, and one of Henry's paintings—for the last three years he had been creating large, wildly colorful paintings, an attempt to express the complexity of his emotions—leaned up against the rear bumper, as if for sale. As if some passerby would ignore the carnage of the garage door and inquire about the availability of this cool painting. Nigel told me his car was still running, its radio blaring. Overall, not the update from New Orleans I wanted to receive. The only thing missing from the picture was Henry. Nigel said he had no idea where Henry was. I asked him to please turn the car off and take the keys. I told him I would handle everything else. Nigel was patient and empathetic. But it wasn't as if he didn't have responsibilities of his own. He is a highly regarded transplant doctor at Ochsner and is in charge of their program. He has two young kids and never seemed to judge Henry. He visited Henry when he was hospitalized at Ochsner and has always been there for him. Henry befriended his two young sons when they moved next door to us. Henry's kindness with his sons, I think, had created a fan in Nigel. Throughout all of Henry's craziness, he never judged or tried to shame any of us. On the contrary.

Having a son suffering from severe mental illness is hard for everyone, especially our closest friends. They had no idea what we were going through, and yet, they wanted to be there for us. They didn't know what to say, so they said nothing. They loved us but didn't know how to help. There was nothing they could do or say that would help us. What they didn't know was that just being there and listening to our chaos was helpful. Just letting us be sad for the life we no longer had was enough. We were often looking for that shoulder to cry on. I am more an open book than Heidi is. I'll say anything to anyone. Heidi has a tough time being that open, often suffering in silence. Her friends wanted to help, but she was incapable of letting them. This is a self-fulfilling prophecy, and her spiral deepened. Heidi is loved by many. For every person I called a friend, Heidi has five. But she felt alone and isolated. She wanted to let people in but felt judged and ashamed. She was convinced that when she went out and saw people that they would scatter, flee. I felt bad for Heidi, but there was nothing I could do to convince her otherwise. We talked about it at therapy with Andre, and I know that helped a little. All of her friends stuck with her, and, though she tried to distance herself, they would not allow it. Another thing to be grateful for.

But at that moment, I was not grateful for anything. I had a garage door that was open to the street. More importantly,

I had a missing son clearly in psychosis. So, I did what I do. I got to work. I called Cecile at work and asked if she could get her unit to look for Henry and take him back to the hospital. I asked her to make sure they took him to University Hospital, so he could get back into Dr. Weiss' care. I then called Serena to make sure they knew to put him on the Tulane floor. Unbelievably, all of this happened as planned. I also called my contractor to see if he could board up our garage. After all, an open garage in New Orleans is an open invitation. He was also able to help. Yet another person now added to the circle of people who knew about Henry—though at this point it was not a well-kept secret. I'm sure we were talked about at dinner tables around the city. While that burdened Heidi, it had little effect on me. I had bigger problems, and I was starting to learn that hiding from them never served me well. I had finally accepted that I had a sick son. Better late than never.

chapter 27

THE GIRL AND THE GOAT

Henry was now under the care of Dr. Weiss and her team. He had continuity of care for the first time, something missing in modern medicine. When I was a child, I had the same pediatrician my whole life. He knew me and knew my medical history. My kids had the same. But medicine has changed dramatically, and, today, this kind of continuity of care is rare. Yet, it's essential in successfully treating mental health. It was important to have a doctor who knew Henry personally, someone who knew his rhythms, his troubles, and his medical history. This was the first time Henry had had such a luxury.

While I am generally a hopeful person, the weight of Henry's disease was starting to chip away at me. I always felt that Henry would be able to get his disease under control. He needed to accept his diagnosis. Heidi and I had already reached that point of acceptance. Henry, it turned out, needed more persuasion. He allowed us to visit him, which we did every day. He realized that if he wanted to stay out of the hospital he needed to stay on his medications, and, while he was still not willing to admit he was sick, he didn't want to end up back in the psych ward. From everything Henry was saying, we were beginning to believe that he had a shot at some sort of normal life. He wanted to return to school and had only two more semesters to go. He was twenty-five, soon to be twenty-six, and wanted to get on with things. He wanted to be a teacher or to work with kids in some capacity. After he was released, he re-enrolled at UNO and was happy to be in school again. He seemed to be taking his medication, as he was stable and less angry. He was living in the apartment connected to Kate's house. A's and Aces was kind enough to take him back, and, to help them out, I again donated cash to cover his salary. He loved working with the kids. That spring was pretty uneventful, which is to say it was a great spring. Living in a world of constant chaos means that any semblance of calm or normalcy is a welcome relief. Of course, we were still waiting for the next shoe to drop. But for now, everyone had their shoes on. Life's tender mercies. Hashtag blessed.

Life went on, and summer was fast approaching. Henry was taking summer school classes, so he could graduate in December and decided to miss Watervale yet again. Nothing I said could change his mind. He just didn't want to go. I'm not sure if he didn't want to go because he didn't want to talk to others about his setbacks or if he was just punishing us, as he knew we loved being there as a family. Either way, he wasn't going.

Patti was living in Chicago. She had graduated from Trinity College in Connecticut in 2012 and moved to New York. In New York City, she worked for a publicist who specialized in design clients. She lived with two high school friends from New Orleans. She had lots of Trinity friends living in the city as well. Patti was a diligent worker and very smart but never really fell in love with New York. After three years, she decided to escape. She had spent three summers waitressing at Watervale, so she had a lot of friends living in Chicago. When one of them told her she was looking for a roommate, Patti jumped at the chance. Only one problem: she had no job. When one of her bigger clients found out, they offered to create a job for her at their showroom in Chicago. Typical Patti. She is such a hard worker and so smart and attentive, who would not want her as an employee. Off she went to Chicago, primed for a new adventure.

Patti, by living thousands of miles away, had not had to deal as directly with Henry's illness. I was glad she had escaped the chaos and had been able to carve out a life of her own. Before we arrived at Watervale, we always stayed for a couple of days with Heidi's parents first, just outside of Chicago. I had business in Chicago, so I told Patti I would come up a day early and take her to dinner wherever she wanted to go. She chose The Girl and the Goat, a popular restaurant and a hard reservation. She was able to get us in at 7 p.m. I met her at a nearby rooftop bar after she left work. We had a cocktail and caught up before heading to the restaurant. They sat us right away, brought us water and some menus. As we were looking at the menu my phone rang. It was Kate.

"What's up?" I said. "I'm at dinner with Patti. Excited to see you and Mom tomorrow."

"Dad, Henry's on the front porch with just a shirt and no pants," she explained.

"What? Really? Have you called Mom?"

"Yep. She said to call you."

Great. I was miles away at dinner with my oldest child. I told Kate I would handle it. As I hung up, Patti asked me what was going on. I told her about Henry, and I could see the concern coming over her face like a summer storm coming down the street. Before I could offer Patti any words of comfort, I started to feel dizzy. I thought I was going to faint. That was the last thought I had before I fainted.

Fainting is surreal. When you finally come to, it is like being woken from a deep sleep. Disoriented. Not sure where you are. The first time this happened I was playing tennis indoors at the Hilton in New Orleans. We were playing doubles, and I went up to hit an overhead. When I came down, I thought my partner had hit me on the back of my leg with his racquet. When I saw this could not have been possible, I thought maybe a ball had hit me. When I took my first step, I knew something was wrong. What I later learned was the sound I heard was the sound of my calf muscle popping. Not fun and extremely painful. I limped over to the side and sat down. One of the players on the next court was a doctor. He kept moving my foot and asking if that hurt. Each movement hurt a lot. That was the last thing I remember. The next thing I knew I was prone on the court, and ten people were looking at me. My first thought was, "Oh my god, I forgot to wear pants."

After about a minute I realized where I was. The facility made me leave in an ambulance and get tests done at the hospital. They did a brain scan, and it came back 100% that I do have a brain. My family proven wrong yet again. I had suffered from a vasovagal syncope, causing my body to shut down. It is what the body does when experiencing physical or emotional pain that overwhelms it. My body was rebooting, and, luckily, it was only about a sixty-second reboot. It must be terrifying for those with you at the time, but I wouldn't know about that. I was passed out.

Waking up in a crowded Chicago restaurant is a tad unsettling. My first thought was that I had actually wet my pants. My crotch area was soaked, why else would all these people be staring at me? After about a minute, I started regaining my senses, and my eyes found Patti, who looked as if she had just witnessed her favorite doll being tossed out the window. But the waitress was closer, right in my face as if her proximity could will me back to the land of the living. Everyone involved thought I was having a heart attack, and they had already called an ambulance. I explained this had happened before, and it was a vasovagal reaction to some disturbing news I had just received. They had no idea what a vasovagal reaction was and were more concerned that I not die in the middle of their popular restaurant with the hard reservation. No one needed that Yelp review of the guy who had wet his pants and died on a Thursday night. While waiting for the ambulance, I was able to talk to Patti for a second and calm her down.

"I'm fine," I reassured her, "This has happened before. I just heard about Henry, and it got to me. No heart attack. I'm fine. By the way, why are my pants wet? Please tell me I did not pee in my pants?" A question you never want to have to ask your daughter. She laughed. "They were dousing you with water trying to revive you. Must have dripped down your pants. You did not piss yourself." She was now laughing hysterically in between trying to get it together.

The ambulance showed up, and two paramedics came over to ask me some questions. They were concerned about my heart, and, though it was indeed broken, it was not anything they could fix. I told them that it was a vasovagal reaction, and, while they knew what that was, they weren't ready to give up the heart attack theory. It probably did not help that once they got me out of the restaurant, I vomited. We hadn't ordered yet, so it wasn't much. But I wasn't in great shape, and Patti was no longer laughing. She was worried about her dad. The medics asked her if she wanted to ride up front with them to the hospital. She readily agreed. I begged them not to tell her the heart attack theory, as I knew it was wrong. I knew exactly what had happened. On the way to the hospital, I overheard the discussion with the doctors in the emergency room telling the paramedics not to give me nitroglycerine. Any treatment could wait as I was in no pain, and my vitals were fine. Meanwhile up front the paramedic totally disregarded my explicit instructions and informed Patti that I had probably had a heart attack. We got to the hospital where I was rushed right into the cardiac wing of the emergency room.

I have been to plenty of emergency rooms, mostly with Henry as a kid. One time it was from getting popcorn stuck up his nose. Heidi and the kids were at the movies, and Henry thought he had popcorn stuck up his nose—at least until he saw the pair of tweezers the doctors were wielding. The popcorn magically disappeared. Then, there was the time he broke his arm playing football the day before his eighth-grade trip to North Carolina. We were there for two hours until his arm was set, and a temporary cast put on. That meant he could not go on his trip. He was pissed. He yelled, "I just want to kill myself!" Well, there went another hour as one psychiatrist after another had to make sure he wasn't serious. He wasn't.

As I entered the emergency room, I expected to wait. I soon discovered that if they even *think* you're having heart conditions you go to the front of the line. As I was being wheeled in, I kept trying to tell everyone I was fine. The paramedics even agreed that I was looking much better. At which point the nurse says, "He looked worse?" Gee, thanks. Once they determined I was not having a heart attack, they let me see Patti.

"Dad, are you okay? You scared the hell out of me. They said you were having a heart attack."

"Well, don't believe everything you hear," I replied. "I'm fine. One more test, and they told me I could leave."

At this point it was already ten, and none of us had eaten. I told Patti to go home, and I would be fine. She was worried and reluctant to leave, but I insisted and by eleven she left. It was a Thursday night, the downtown Chicago emergency room was packed, so I was kept on a gurney in the hall. Looking around I noticed all the other "patients." Many were handcuffed to their beds. Many looked unshowered. Many were talking to themselves and very little of it made sense. I had a front row seat to some very disturbed people, albeit from a new vantage point. The irony was not lost on me. I called Heidi. She was waiting.

"You gave Patti quite the scare," she said. "She was freaking out when she first called. Are you okay?"

"I'm fine," I replied. "It's just like the time I passed out at the Hilton. It's a major inconvenience, but I am fine. How's Henry?"

"He's okay. He's a little manic, but we leave tomorrow. I think he'll be fine until we get back. I think he was just trying to push Kate's buttons." He was always good at that! While I was relieved, I was pissed that I had let Henry ruin my night with Patti. As far away as Patti was, it turns out, it was not far enough.

Watervale was its usual joy for all of us, minus the fact that we were without Henry and missing him. While this disappointed me, it really threw Heidi for a loop. She loved her family, and Henry's absence was excruciating for her. At least the girls were there. We were learning to be a family of four. It seemed Henry was done with us and wanted his space. Given the fact that we had him hospitalized numerous times, it was going to take a long time for him to let us back in. In the meantime, we were learning to be happy with what we had.

Upon our return, Henry seemed to be doing better.

Maybe he was right: maybe we *were* part of the problem. We gave him his space. He continued to work at A's and Aces as well as delivering food for various services. He was also playing poker at Harrah's Casino downtown. And he was winning more than he was losing. Things were so stable that I decided to throw more chaos into the mix. I told Heidi that I wanted a second dog. Heidi looked at me as if I were a Martian.

"Are you crazy? As if we don't have enough to worry about? You must be smoking something stronger than pot if you think we are getting another dog." But I was ready for precisely this reaction. I had even rehearsed my response.

"Heidi, we love Bella so much. I think we should get her a friend to play with. I want a brown one. They would look so cute together. I think it will make things easier, not harder." Heidi did love Bella, and I managed to win her over. So, right after Thanksgiving I drove to Missouri to pick up Bodie, our little brown puppy, and Bella's new sister. Turns out she was the runt of the litter and scared of her own shadow. But she was cute, and Bella loved having a playmate.

Her own shadow was not the only thing Bodie was afraid of. Bodie was scared of Henry, as well. And as much as he tried, she kept running away from him. Henry, undeterred, eventually won Bodie over. He would come by just to see the dogs. He loved them, and they loved him. He would get on all fours, his hair in his eyes as the dogs treated him as one of their own. I smiled, listening to his laugh as the dogs licked him. The look on his face playing with those dogs reminded me of his days jumping on the trampoline. Not a care in the world for a happy little boy blessed by life. The way his life could have been. The way his life should have been.

chapter 28

SEATTLE

By December 2019, Henry had enough credits to graduate from UNO. This was something I never thought would happen. A tribute to his remarkable perseverance. Just as he was on a tennis court, Henry was a fighter. He had graduated from college. I was proud of him and told him so. He waved me off as if my opinion did not matter. He was still angry with me for all the hospitalizations. I didn't let the moment pass. I wanted to make a big deal about this. Like it or not, Henry was going to get validation from me. We took him to his favorite vegan restaurant to celebrate. And while he acted like he didn't care, I suspect he did.

Not only had Henry graduated, but he had also quickly found a job in Seattle, Washington. Neither Heidi nor I was too happy that Seattle was 2,617 miles away. But we were both happy that he found a job he liked. He was hired as a Lower School P.E. teacher for the Jewish Day School. The irony was hard to miss. My atheist kid, who had fought me every Sunday morning to avoid going to Sunday School, was teaching at a Jewish Day school. Even he had to laugh. He was supposed to start the first week of January, and he planned on driving to Seattle. He wanted to do the forty-hour drive in three days.

He would leave the day after Christmas. He also needed to find a place to live. The head of the school had a small Airbnb that he let Henry use while he looked for an apartment.

Henry was excited to be out on his own, and, while Heidi and I were nervous, we were excited as well. My brother always used to say that if you wanted self-esteem, do self-esteeming things. This was a step in the right direction. We were proud of him and more importantly, we could see he was proud of himself. He had been to hell and back, several times in fact, and he had persevered.

His leaving was emotional for Heidi and me. Heidi, who wears her emotions on her sleeves, cried as she told him goodbye. She also demanded her hug. Henry gratefully obliged. My turn. Henry hated it when I told him I loved him. I don't know why. Maybe he thought that a father who would hospitalize his son against his wishes didn't actually love him. Who knows? What I did know was that every time I told him I loved him it made him visibly uncomfortable. I didn't care. I hugged him and told him I loved him, how proud I was of him. I hoped these words penetrated the hard shell he surrounded himself with. My hope was that he heard those words and believed them. My guess was he was not ready to forgive. I knew deep down that Henry loved me. At this moment, it was very deep down. However, he was excited to be leaving, so he threw us a bone and smiled. "I'll call when I get there." And then he disappeared down the street.

With our tracking device still hidden in his car, we were able to follow him on his road trip. Having a kid with mental illness, you're never fully relaxed. No matter how quiet things are, there is that expectation of chaos. After a while you begin to get used to it, like wearing weights around your ankles when walking. It's not until the weights are removed that you feel the lightness. I stood a little straighter and hoped that with Henry's job, and with him being far away from us, maybe our family could begin to experience a new era.

Henry arrived in Seattle and actually *did* call us. He soon found an apartment near his work that was affordable and began his new life as a P.E. teacher. All seemed to be going well. Still unable to believe that things could be so good, I would follow Henry through his car to see if he was really going to work. He was. I began to relax. I watched his daily routine from afar thanks to technology. Then one Saturday, a month after he began his job, he took the car on a long drive about sixty miles south of Seattle. It was curious to me, and my brain went into overdrive. I, of course, assumed there was a casino there. Then the car stayed there overnight. And the next night. And the night after that.

I had always been able to track his car, but I never considered tracking his phone. Perhaps that would have been the smarter move. Where the hell was Henry? I began sleuthing. I drilled down closer and saw that the car was near a used car lot. But how could he sell the car when the title was in my name? Turns out, of course, that makes no difference in the often-sketchy used car world. Sure enough, three days later the tracker went silent and that was the last I heard from the car. It was as if this blue, 2015 Honda Pilot was pissed at me too and had decided to quit talking. How was I going to bring this up to Henry without blowing my cover? Did it even matter anymore? I didn't want him to know. What little trust I had with him would be destroyed. I was paralyzed and unsure of what to do. So, I did what I said I wouldn't do. I called him.

Subtlety has never been my strong suit. Yet, I was going to need to figure out a way to bring up the car. Heidi was worried that we were in the beginning of another manic episode. I wasn't sure she was wrong. I called him, and he picked up. I started asking a bunch of questions. How was work? What did he do on weekends? Where did he park the car? As I said, subtlety, not a strong suit. "Why do you care about the car? What difference does it make to you? It's my car."

"Technically, it's still registered in my name."

That did it. Now, he was pissed. I'd pulled out the money card, and he hated it when I did that.

"If it's your car, how come I was able to sell it?"

There it was. Mystery solved. As soon as he had said it, he realized the opening it had given me.

"What?" I asked in a bewildered tone. "You sold the car? Why did you do that? *How* did you do that?"

Now, he was getting smug. "Wasn't hard. They just gave me a little less money for it. It was my car, and I didn't need it. I could use the extra cash, so I sold it. Get over it."

Now, *I* was pissed. This was usually the point where his disrespect triggered my deepest insecurities, and I would lash out in return. I had done it in Florida with Henry, and I knew it wouldn't end well. For maybe the first time in my life, I kept my cool. I didn't take the bait. Instead, I deflected. "Well, how are you going to get around?"

"I can walk. I live close to school, and I walk everywhere."

He calmed down, and we were able to have a relatively peaceful discussion. At least I knew what had happened. Clearly, in a more manic state, he had decided to get rid of the car. I knew that he had sold it cheaply, and the dealmaker in me was upset. But in the big picture of all the money we had spent on Henry, this was a drop in the bucket. And at least he had been honest with me, and I hadn't lost my shit and allowed the conversation to devolve into the heated back and forth we were both capable of. I took the win and left it alone. I was getting better at this. And Heidi, listening to the whole conversation, was proud of me. I chalked it up as a victory and let it go. I was sure Henry was doing the same.

Maybe I was finally learning. Maybe all those years of therapy were paying off. Maybe we were finding our way to the good side of this thing. Maybe we were waking up from our nightmare. It was February 2020, and things were looking pretty good. Then Covid-19 struck.

chapter 29

THE PUNCH

Covid-19 tipped over many people's lives. Henry was no exception. By March of 2020, America was shutting down. Some of the first institutions to close were schools. The Jewish Day School of Seattle sent everyone home, with the idea that classes would be held remotely. It's one thing to teach math remotely; it's a whole other matter to do P.E. remotely. I'm not even sure how this could be done. I could imagine him on a Zoom call with ten-year-olds. "Rachel, that's not much of a push-up." "Jonathan, if you don't think I see those Tootsie Roll wrappers, you're wrong."

What I'm sure about is that the disruption to Henry's routine was not helpful to his mental health. A study released by the World Health Organization (WHO) said that global prevalence of anxiety and depression increased by 25% in the first year of the pandemic. This can be explained by many factors, not the least of which would be social isolation. Henry was not good in unstructured environments, and this was the mother of all unstructured environments. Living alone in a 700-square-foot studio apartment in a city where he knew no one took its toll on Henry. He began to call home frequently and complain about his boredom. He thought that Covid-19 was most likely a scam. I could see that his conspiracy theories, especially in left-leaning Seattle, were not going to be well-received. Both Heidi and I encouraged him to come back and "work" from home. I offered to pay for the ticket. Unbelievably, he agreed.

As soon as Henry came home, I guessed his password and enabled the Find My iPhone feature on his phone, so I could track his location. Once again, my control issues were taking center stage and feeling that I could track him gave me comfort. I know I would have been happier if I could just let go of my need to control. But it was hard to do. So, we tracked his phone instead of the car he no longer had.

We could tell things were not good. His appearance was growing increasingly disheveled, and his Zoom calls with the staff at the Jewish Day School had all but disappeared. When home, he would stay in his room for hours on end, occasionally coming downstairs to pick fights with Heidi and me. Heidi was impossible to bait. She would not allow her love and devotion to Henry to be compromised. And her calm demeanor made her seemingly impenetrable to his taunts. But I knew better. She suffered in silence, after being called a bitch and far worse by a more and more manic Henry. Feeling protective of her, I would jump into the fray. That only caused more insults to rain down. In my eagerness to protect her, I was, in fact, making things much worse. Especially since she didn't need or want my "protection." Heidi and I began to fight, which I think Henry secretly enjoyed. As bad as Henry was, Heidi wanted him around. I didn't and after three weeks, I asked Henry to go back to Seattle. Heidi hated this idea, but Henry was eager to oblige. So, now I had a wife who was pissed off at me and a son flying 2,617 miles away in a state of mind that was unraveling.

Henry called five days later. Heidi and I knew he was in psychosis when he told us he had destroyed his passport and his driver's license. He rambled on about the government getting their hands on his papers. I never really got to the bottom of that. Here's what I did know: my son increasingly looked like the Unabomber and had no ID to prove he wasn't. There was nothing I could do about the manic state. There was no way he was being allowed on an airplane.

Fortunately, Louisiana was one of the first states to establish digital driver's licenses. Henry had one on his phone. Thus, while he could not travel out of the country (a good thing), he could still get home if they accepted the digital license. I explained he could work from home and living with us would save him money on food and other things. It was early May, and school was ending anyway. Henry agreed and was able to use his digital ID to get through security. I can only imagine the trip home. Talking to security, explaining that the ID on your phone was all you had. And while in a manic state. And the flight attendants. The stories they must have about this strange kid with the hoodie.

I picked Henry up at the airport. He was dressed in his usual outfit of sweatpants and a sweatshirt. His hair was dirty, and he smelled like he hadn't showered in a while. When I asked about work, he confessed that he had been fired about a month ago. Henry told me that, to make extra money, he had sent his students flyers about teaching tennis. This earned him a warning from the head of school. When he sent out another batch of flyers, he was fired. On the ride home from the airport, I realized Henry was in a manic state. He was speaking rapidly, sentence after sentence with no real punctuation between any of them. His eyes darted from object to object. Heidi noticed it as soon as he walked through the front door. Once the manic cycle started, it was hard for Henry to turn it off. It usually ended when his mania morphed into psychosis, requiring hospitalization. Luckily, he was home where we could keep an eye on him.

Mother's Day 2020 was the day it all blew up. The preceding days had been getting worse and worse. We reached the point on Friday afternoon that we felt we needed another Order of Protective Custody. Our fourth. Every time we got one of these, we always hoped we would not need it. This time was no different. He already hated us for the previous times, and one more from us might send him away forever. The pain and anguish of this was soul-crushing. I was reminded of those old Tarzan movies when some guy gets caught in quicksand. He slowly sinks until he disappears from sight. Here I was jumping in the quicksand myself, hoping I would be able to find a way out. A tree branch. A lucky soul wandering by. Instead, I got the paper from the coroner, came home, and hoped he would get better. Not much of a plan.

That weekend was tough as Henry slipped deeper and deeper into psychosis. By Saturday night we knew we would have to use the protective order. Heidi never wanted to make the decision whether we should use it. She always left it to me. She knew I would make the tough call when necessary, and it was quickly becoming necessary. Henry was not sleeping at all, and Heidi and I only slightly better. At 7 a.m. Sunday morning, I heard the front door close. He was on the loose. I quickly got dressed and went outside. I could see him a block away. Unfortunately, I could hear him, as well. To call it singing would be like calling the sounds of seals barking at each other singing. It was closer to screaming, and I was concerned that the neighbors would soon have the police on their way. I ran to Henry. "Hey, Henry. Where are you going?"

"I'm going to visit Kate."

"Kate is the other direction," I said as gently as I could. "Why don't you come home, and we can call Kate. I'm worried that the neighbors will call the police, and you'll end up back in the hospital."

Actually, I was hoping a neighbor *would* call the police and he *would* end up back in the hospital.

"Come on. Let's just go home, and we can talk there," I begged.

"Okay," he replied, and I turned around to lead him home. When I turned back around to see if he was following me, the only thing I saw was a huge fist coming right at my face. Before I had time to react, he connected with the left side of my eye.

I have only been in one fight in my life. Being small in high school, I learned to avoid fights. Once in ninth grade, another small kid, Chris, felt that he could get some street cred by picking a fight with me. Not exactly David versus Goliath. More like David versus David. And while I was small, I was fast and scrappy. I had never been much of a fighter, but the fear of being ridiculed by the sharks of ninth grade was motivating. My adrenaline was rushing, and I could hear my heart beating. Chris was unprepared for the fury of a scared, cornered ninth grader. I got him to the ground and held him in a tight hold until he started yelling for help. I let him up and moved on. Though victorious, I did not feel like it. My friends were all patting my back, but I just wanted to disappear. Fighting had never been my thing. Even wrestling in high school, I had lacked that killer instinct. I was fast and strong, so I usually won. Yet, when I came up against people who were killers, I always lost.

In all my years, I had avoided being hit hard and never with a closed fist. It hurts. You see the fights in movies with guys getting hit hard, and they seem like they're being hit with a pillow. This punch felt more like a brick. Stars exploded in my head. But I did not go down! Reeling and confused, I was still upright. Barely. One more punch and I'd be done. I was ready for the taking. I could feel the blood running down my face, and, when I put a hand to my throbbing head, it came away wet, sticky, and bright red. Maybe it was the sight of the blood, maybe it was the fright of what he had just done.

Whatever it was, Henry seemed repulsed and scared. For a few seconds that felt like minutes, our eyes locked. In that brief time, it was like I was looking into his soul. I could see his compassion and his disgust at what he had done. But what hurt more than the punch was the shame I saw in those eyes. And then he was gone.

I yelled after him. Henry never turned back. We both knew what my next call would be. I called the police and told them I had a 72-hour hold and needed my son picked up. They asked where he was, and I told them I didn't know but was sure he was close by. He was on foot and how far could he go. A police officer showed up, asking a lot of questions. Looking at me with blood caked to the side of my face, a gash clearly visible, he wanted to know if Henry was violent. When I answered no and said Henry would not hurt anyone, the cop laughed. "It doesn't look that way to me."

"I'm his dad, and there are plenty of other issues," I tried to explain. "He'd never hurt anyone else and was scared at what he'd done to me. He's a sweet kid who is having a psychotic episode."

"We'll do our best to bring him peacefully," the officer said. "I'm just concerned what might happen if he resists."

"He won't resist." I was hoping I was right.

My next call was to Dave, a good friend and a great plastic surgeon. He was also married to a plastic surgeon, Ruth, who was slowing down her career to focus on her painting—a true artist with a brush as well as a knife. It was about 9 a.m. when

I called Dave, who answered right away. He was in the car with Ruth, on their way to a restaurant near me for a Mother's Day breakfast. This call was tough for me since I was having to air our family's dirty secret to yet another friend, and, while everyone knew of Henry's condition, no one person knew everything. Reluctantly, I told them what had happened and asked if I could meet them at the restaurant so they could assess the damage. They were nice enough to agree. I was getting ready to go when they called. It turned out the restaurant was closed, so they asked me to take a picture of my face and text it over. Thirty seconds later my cell phone rang. It was Ruth. "Tripp, this is bad. You're going to need stitches. Can you meet us at Dave's office at ten?" I did. Eighteen stitches later I was sewn up and back at home. The hunt for Henry was still ongoing. I learned he had seen a police car and bolted. He was in our neighborhood at least. I was able to track his phone, but it was not moving. It was near our house, but the location was general and not specific. The next call was from the mother of a friend of Henry's. "Tripp, Henry just jumped off our roof into the pool. He was soaking wet, so we gave him some clothes. He's a bit incoherent. He just left, but we were worried and wanted to call to let you know."

"Thanks. We're worried as well. Sorry about that. He's not well right now. Thanks again." And yet another person getting a peek behind the curtain. Our dark little secret was escaping around town. But how could Henry have been over there when the phone said he was just a few blocks away? That made no sense. I was confused. I later learned that while being chased, he crawled under a house and left his phone there by accident. He was never able to accurately describe which house. But I'm pretty sure there is a perfectly good iPhone under a house in the 1800 block of Calhoun Street.

Finally, the doorbell rang, and it was the police. They had found Henry around the corner, and, when they called his name, he came peacefully. He was in the back of the police car, but he would not look at me. I suspect he was ashamed of having hit me. He wasn't screaming at me or calling me names. It was as if he knew where he was going and had accepted his fate. Like the man before a firing squad who knows the end is near. They told us they were taking him to the University Medical Center. I rushed down there, so they knew to admit him to the Tulane wing if at all possible. Fate was smiling on us, as there was room in this wing, and Henry was admitted. As this was during Covid, we were not allowed to visit. It was just as well. Both Henry and I needed time to heal.

chapter 30

BRIGHTQUEST

Henry was in the hospital for two weeks. They put him on medication, and he slept. He met with doctors and therapists and accepted his confinement with grace. It was as if he finally felt safe in a hospital and wanted to stay. Maybe punching me was a wake-up call for Henry. Heidi and I were busy trying to find Henry a long-term solution, a place where he could go once he was released from the hospital. While Henry was not fighting his treatment, we knew that getting him into a long-term program would be a challenge. Threading that needle of a place that treated bipolar disorder *and* was a community Henry would agree to become a part of was tricky. There were many treatment centers, but most were addiction centers that treated mental illness secondarily. We needed a place that primarily treated mental illness. We found the perfect one: BrightQuest Treatment Center in San Diego. BrightQuest began in 1979 as a therapeutic space for individuals suffering from complex mental illness. It was founded with a strong Native American tradition of individuals going on a vision quest as part of their healing process. Henry, who was into alternative theories of mind expansion, was going to love that. BrightQuest was started by Moira Fitzpatrick when she began suffering from symptoms of schizophrenia. She recovered and went on to live a productive life. Forty-one years later, I was hoping BrightQuest could do for Henry what it had done for many others. Henry was reluctant at first but finally agreed to give it a try.

We called BrightQuest and arranged for an interview with Henry. We knew this would go well, as Henry had always been compliant when confined to a hospital. It was usually once he was out that he became more volatile and unpredictable. Henry came through his interview just fine. Then, Heidi and I were interviewed. They had space for Henry and wanted to talk to us about the financial commitment. BrightQuest ran on the assumption you would be there a while. The first step was called Intensive Residential. That was $30,000 a month. The next phase was Community Based Residential. That was $15,000 a month. The phase after that was Semi-Independent Living. That was $7,500 a month. You get the idea. This treatment would run us over $100,000. That figure was astonishing to me. Insurance would cover very little of it, so it was mostly on us. The mental illness treatment game is stacked against those who can't afford it. The unfairness of it all is apparent. I was lucky I could afford it and, given our desperation, would have gladly paid more if there was a guarantee it would work. But of course, these types of treatment centers don't come with guarantees. I agreed to pay for it and hoped it would work. In the meantime, our biggest concern was actually getting Henry there.

Having gone down this path before, we knew we had to go straight from the hospital to the airport and hope Henry would get on the plane with us. This was May of 2020, still the early days of Covid, and traveling by airplane was awful. Masks were mandatory, and airlines were short staffed. Henry, being the generous kid he was, had requested we bring some extra shoes and socks for some of the other patients. With apparel in tow, we picked Henry up at the hospital. After leaving his gifts with the nurse who brought him down to the car, we drove straight to the airport, hoping that Henry would not change his mind. Lines were short, and we managed to get through security without too much hassle. Given the fact that Henry was going to another treatment center, the hospital had released him, even though he was still a little manic. This made traveling even more difficult. We had to change planes in Houston, and watching a manic Henry wander through Hobby Airport was an odyssey. It was like he was four years old again. A boy in a supermarket wanting to put his hands on every pop tart within his reach. I needed to keep an eye on him without it being seen as surveillance.

We finally made it to San Diego. The airport was nearly empty. It reminded me of those deserted towns in the old westerns. An occasional passenger would hurry by like tumbleweed. It was eerie. At the Hertz counter, we were literally the only people other than the guy behind it. He was so happy to see another human that he let us have any car we wanted. Henry wanted a BMW, so that's what we chose. We drove to the hotel and checked in. I informed the person checking us in that we would not want housekeeping services. I wanted our privacy given Henry's state of mind. The person checking us in laughed. "That's a good thing as we only clean rooms when people check out. You will need to bring your trash to the lobby to throw it away. Also, no breakfast, just a box with a roll and some fruit." Traveling during Covid was indeed strange.

We had a bedroom suite, with a pull-out couch. We wanted to be between Henry and the exit, so we took the pull-out couch. Someone had to play warden. We had an inmate who was known to escape. It had been a long day by the time we got to bed. We woke up the next morning ready for our intake interview. Henry met with the counselors as we met with the finance person. While I was learning just what this intervention would cost, Henry was being his manic self and not endearing himself to the counselors. The plan was to go back to the hotel, then drop him off the next morning, catch a flight to Seattle, pack up his things, and head home. That was the plan. And like all our plans, it did not go as planned.

On the way back to the hotel, I received a call that Henry was too manic to start the program. I was in the car with both Heidi and Henry, so I asked if I could call back when I got back to the hotel. When we got back, I told Heidi. She was visibly upset. She was beat and ready to admit defeat. She had gone fifteen rounds and had nothing left. She held back the tears for Henry's sake, but I could see the sadness. Her eyes bore right through my heart. I knew I had to do something.

I left the hotel for a walk and called the head counselor at BrightQuest. She reiterated her concern that Henry was still too manic for the program. She said we would need to find a hospital for him until he became less manic. I felt like I was in one of those movies where you see the man dangling from a rope, and the rope begins to fray. In about one minute, the rope will rip, sending the man plummeting to his death. Heidi and I were hanging by a thread. I felt that putting Henry in the hospital at this point would put all of our plans at risk. I asked if we could have one more day of rest and medication to see if he would settle down. She agreed. The rope stopped fraying, at least for a moment. I went back inside and told Heidi who was relieved but still concerned. All of this chaos had beaten any optimism out of her. She only felt despair. She wanted to be positive, but, after all life had thrown at her, it was hard. I held her tight and whispered that everything would work out. I almost believed my lie.

Henry fell asleep at 7 p.m. that night. My sleep was harder to come by. Even with a Klonopin, I had a rough night. I awoke early the next morning, and Henry was still sleeping. I snuck out to not wake either him or Heidi and went for a run to clear my head. When I got back Heidi was awake, but Henry was still sleeping. We had set our meeting for 9 a.m. I knew that sleep was the great elixir—that the more the better—so I called the office and moved our meeting back until one. He woke up at ten, and the mania seemed to be gone. He was grumpy but not manic. The day was looking up.

It was a sunny day in San Diego with the temperature in the eighties and no humidity. The kind of day we may get ten of in New Orleans all year. It was as if the gods were smiling. It is amazing how the weather can change everything. Heidi went from dark to bright, and, for the first time in a long time, I felt that everything would be fine. We drove Henry to his meeting and went for a walk in the neighborhood hoping that they would see the Henry we saw. They did. He would be admitted the next day. I changed our flights once again and made sure the hotel could take us another night. Now, all I had to do was keep Henry from changing his mind. Another Klonopin and another sleepless night later, Henry was ready for check in at BrightQuest. I think he was as tired of all of this as we were. We drove to BrightQuest in complete silence, trying our best not to say anything for fear it would change his mind.

Henry's wallet had fallen under the seat the night before. I found it and kept it, not wanting him to have access to any money. When it came time to leave him, he wanted to know where his wallet was. I played dumb and looked for it but no luck. I told him I would find it and send it but that for now he did not need it. BrightQuest also had a no cell phone rule. They took his cellphone until he "earned" it back. This was hard for Henry, and I was worried it would be the proverbial straw. The fact that a cute girl was checking him in was helpful. Before his disease, Henry was a bit of a ladies' man. Tall, dark, and handsome. But his illness had made dating impossible. It seemed obvious now that Henry still liked cute girls, so he kept his irascibility to a minimum. And just like that we were giving him a hug and saying goodbye.

We got in the car to head to the airport. That was when Heidi broke down. Tears flowed down her face. It was the culmination of four long days on the heels of six long years. It was as if she could finally cry for the son she loved so dearly but could never help. She cried like I had never seen. And while I'm sure it was cathartic for her, it confused me. Why wasn't she relieved? Why wasn't she happy that we were finally on a good path? Was I missing something? I was. In my zeal to be a fixer, I had rarely stopped to consider the pain Heidi had lived with. The loss of one son and the mental unraveling of another. These were the tears for a life she never wanted to live. And yet here she was. Tears for all the pain she had lived with. And tears for a seemingly indifferent world. I reached over and held her hand and let her cry. As we drove to the airport hand in hand, tears flowing, my love for Heidi had never been greater.

chapter 31

COMING HOME

Heidi and I arrived in Seattle, rented a car, and drove to another empty hotel in another seemingly deserted town. Our flight back to New Orleans was late the next afternoon, giving us a full day to take care of business. Heidi and I woke up early and headed to Henry's apartment, ready to pack yet another one. Moving Henry out of his apartments was soul crushing, each one worse than the last. This last one was a small but cute studio, located in a nice neighborhood and with a colorful exterior. Going in you could see how exciting Henry's life in Seattle could have been: a job he loved in a place he liked. But like a party girl who didn't age well, the apartment's pretty bones had been destroyed by hard living. Hints of what used to be, broken by what came to be. For every charming detail we could find—like brightly painted cabinetry and tall ceilings—there were piles of dirty laundry and even dirtier dishes. There were no ants this time as there was no food anywhere. The refrigerator was empty yet somehow still filthy. The bathroom was grimy, the shower curtain beginning to mold. The squalor was overwhelming, and sadness overtook us. While the convenience of the UPS store across the street was an unseen benefit, this was a devastating glimpse into an unwell mind. Knowing that it was our son made it even worse. His surfboard stood in the hallway outside his door, a tall and heartbreaking reminder that he was not coming back. It took us only two hours to pack him up this time, as he seemed to have given away many of his things. Or at least they were nowhere to be found. It took another two hours to clean the place so that it looked presentable to the landlord. Yet another lease we would have to buy our way out of. Yet another security deposit gone. Yet another dream squashed by his disease.

Heidi was too busy cleaning to cry. Maybe the day before had dried out all her tears. Maybe the hope of Henry finally getting treatment helped. I knew that sooner or later she would cry over this loss as well. For now, she was like a general in charge of her army of one. Barking orders and taping up boxes for me to carry across the street. Usually, I would balk at being ordered around like that. Today, I did as commanded. By 2 p.m. we were done and ready to head back to the airport to go home. We were physically and emotionally drained and looking forward to a quiet flight back to New Orleans. It was the same Alaska Airlines flight Henry had taken many times. I wondered if the flight attendants were the same, if they had any idea that this frazzled couple were the parents of the frazzled kid they had seen before. We slept the whole way home, exhausted from the stress of the last six days. Exhausted from the stress of the last six years.

BrightQuest was good about staying in touch with us. Every week we'd have a call with Henry's main therapist as well as a call with a therapist of our own. We were now being helped by three different counselors yet felt as alone as ever. Covid had changed everything. Henry had had the audacity to need help in the middle of a worldwide pandemic. The community aspect of BrightQuest had been tapered back to almost nothing. Before Covid, they would hold a family day every other month. Families would come to San Diego to have small group meetings with other families and to see their kids. There would also be a large group meeting where the kids would speak. During Covid all of this was done via Zoom. Meeting three other couples over Zoom and hearing their stories was helpful, yet not quite satisfying—like junk food that fills you up but gives you nothing. Not being able to make those personal connections and have those talks over coffee made the whole thing seem a little cheap. It was like we were getting the "lite" version of this extremely expensive treatment center. Not BrightQuest but LiteQuest. Still, we made do with what we had. After a small meeting with the other parents, we Zoomed in to a larger group. There were already fifty people on the call and finding Henry was like playing Where's Waldo. We finally saw him in the bottom corner of the screen. Henry was there, his picture was on the bottom corner, his image tiny, like a miniature version of our son.

It's hard to get a read on someone over a screen. Hard to hear how they breathe. Hard to see their expressions. The whole interaction is wanting. Yet, it's all we had, and, like a man on a diet, we enjoyed any bite of a cookie we could get.

So, we smiled at each other as we saw his small corner of the screen. We said hi, though I am not sure he heard us, as every other parent was doing the same thing. The definition of a cluster fuck. The meeting started, and it was helpful to hear stories of successes. Henry's was not one of them. Not yet.

Henry was not allowed to speak to us for about a month, so we lived vicariously through the therapists. We were told he was doing well, but it was hard to believe. He was being held at the most restricted level of care, and he was trying to work his way into the next level. It took him about a month, but he accomplished his goal and was moved. Henry was proud of this, and by now he was allowed to talk to us once a week during our therapy sessions with his therapist. Pretty soon he was allowed to talk to us on his own, and, after about three months, we were talking every day. He was limited to twenty minutes a day, but no day went by without a phone call. He seemed happy and finally admitting he had a problem. For the first time ever, I heard him say he had bipolar disorder. This was an enormous step forward.

Whenever we would tell people that Henry had bipolar disorder, they would say, "I hear with drugs, it's manageable." Hell, I used to think so as well. Henry was finally willing to take the drugs but complained they were causing him to gain weight. He had never liked taking the medication, so I dismissed his concerns. Drug companies run ad after ad telling you how helpful these drugs are. These ads all have beautiful people who appear to be thriving. Not overweight. Not shaky.

No apparent side effects, though, if you read the fine print or really listen to the ad, you will see that is far from the truth. Other than weight gain there is akathisia, a form of restlessness. Henry suffered from this, with his leg constantly moving when he sat, like he had a bad case of the shakes. Another is tardive dyskinesia, uncontrollable movements of the jaw, lips, and tongue, which, luckily, Henry did not experience. At least not yet. Then, they give you more drugs for the side effects, which then create more side effects. It is a vicious spiral with no good ending.

Henry was taking Abilify. Heidi and I wanted to get him on the shot you only have to take once a month. This is a much better solution than daily pills, as patients like Henry tend to be noncompliant. The less often they have to take their medication, the better the chance that they'll actually take it. The insurance company, however, did not want to pay for the extra $1,500 a month. It seemed very short-sighted. A stay in a psych ward had to be at least $25,000, and, if getting the medication kept him out of the hospital, it seemed like a smart tradeoff. It took me weeks of fighting with the insurance company, but I was finally able to get it approved. I wondered what happens to those who do not have the means or the knowledge or the sheer will to fight these fights.

At this point, Henry had been at BrightQuest for three months and was living in the community-based residential center. He was doing well, even talking about going to graduate school. He reminded me that I told him the commitment was a month, and he had already been there three months. I told him that I did not think he was ready to leave and encouraged him to keep making a commitment to his improvement. I said that when he could get to the semi-independent living level, we could talk about coming home. He reluctantly agreed. Maybe he really was getting better. Our conversations were certainly warm. We started discussing why and how we had hospitalized him. We were able to have calm discussions about our points of view, and I could tell we were on the right path. By the middle of October, it had been five months, and he was getting close to moving to semi-independent living. He really wanted to be home for Thanksgiving, and we really wanted him home.

I began to talk to his therapist at Tulane, as well as Andre and Serena. Everyone felt he was ready to come home. He had been talking to both his therapist and psychiatrist at Tulane, who agreed as well. BrightQuest was not so sure. They felt that he was doing well, but they wanted him to stay longer and go back to a school near them. BrightQuest wanted to see how he would do under a more supervised regime. This was the first time I had disagreed with them. Despite my respect for the BrightQuest therapists, I found my judgement clouded by my business experience. I do a lot of private equity investing, and, as such, I knew that the mental health field was a place where private equity played. In fact, in 2017 BrightQuest had been purchased by Constellation Behavioral Health, which was a portfolio company of NMS Capital, a private equity shop. I felt that perhaps they were trying to keep Henry longer than was necessary. I was 100% certain that BrightQuest was trying to do what was best for Henry. But even they agreed he was much better and ready for less supervision. They agreed that an outpatient program like Tulane might work; they just felt that it would not hurt to stay another few months.

All of the local health care team disagreed, and Heidi and I wanted Henry home. It had been six months, and the only argument against him coming home was that they were not sure he was ready to go back to school unsupervised. So, we gave them our thirty-day notice and began the process of bringing him home. Henry was excited. He was ready and was more expressive and more himself than he had been in six years. His excitement was contagious, and our excitement grew. He even, on his own, made a dental appointment to get his tooth fixed—which, of course, made Heidi happy. We planned for him to fly home Thursday, November 19, a week before Thanksgiving. We were indeed thankful.

chapter 32

THANKSGIVING

Heidi and I went together to pick Henry up at the New Orleans airport. Too nervous to speak, we drove to the airport in a silence that said everything. It was the kind of nerves you have on a first date. What would he look like? Would he be happy to see us? What should we talk about? We had not seen him in six months since we left him in San Diego. And now he was... what? Cured? Normal? The son his mother and I wanted him to be? The son he was before the disease took hold of him? If so, how would we connect with him, given all the changes he'd been through? What would it be like not to fight at all? To not have the constant arguing about his sleep and his mental health? What would it be like to live without the psychotic episodes? Without the exhaustion of dealing with someone who went from mania to depression like most people changed clothes? And Henry. How would he see us? Would he still see us as villains? Would he know us as the parents who couldn't connect with his troubled mind? Parents who had many times committed him to psych wards of hospitals around the country. Frightening places that no one wants to be in. That no one wants to visit. Could he forgive that?

All these questions raced through my mind as we parked

the car. While I went to meet Henry at baggage claim 4, Heidi waited outside at the curb. As I walked into the airport, I noticed how new and clean it looked. Opened a year earlier, the revamped airport still had that new car feel. Even the baggage claim looked sleek and shiny. The number 4 illuminated in white within a large blue box which sat in the middle of the belt, like an eagle roosting in a tree. I saw Henry before he saw me. Given the holidays, the airport was crowded that day, but it felt like we were the only two people there. A feeling of love and dread washed over me, competing to see which would win. As I looked at him, all my anxieties went away. Love was the clear winner.

He was sitting on a shiny wooden bench, hands on his knees, waiting for the bags to come rolling out. He was dressed in grey baggy sweats, a Chili Peppers sweatshirt, and a baseball cap. He had shaved off all the scruff he usually hid behind. I could actually see his handsome face, which was relaxed, with no signs of the tenseness of the past. His dark brown eyes were soft, and his mouth held the slightest smile.

He had put on weight, at least fifty pounds, which did throw me. Could this really be Henry? It seemed like there were two of him. I had never seen him that heavy. In our phone conversations, Henry had complained that the drugs he was taking caused him to gain weight, but I hadn't been able to picture him. This weight gain was considerable. Yet another side effect. But I was ecstatic to have our Henry back. The fact that there was more of him was of no concern.

I was staring at him as I quickly walked over, unable to get to him fast enough, to hug him and just feel his warm body. As I moved toward him, he turned and looked in my direction, sensing, in some instinctive familial way, that I was there. When he saw me, his eyes lit up as if a dimmed light got turned all the way up. The brightness of those brown eyes warmed me to the core. Then he smiled, ear to ear. It was a smile I hadn't seen in ten years. A genuine smile with no hint of anger or the illness that had haunted him for so long. It cut through all the apprehension of the past, and I grinned back at him with a smile that matched his. Our boy was back. He was here.

By the time I got to Henry, he was standing. I walked up and hugged him for a second longer than he was comfortable. Henry had never been much of a hugger. That didn't stop me. My son was home, and even though he was a lot bigger, he looked good.

"Man, it is great to see you. How many bags are we waiting for?"

"Just one," he said, casting his eyes toward the ground. "Guess you can tell I gained a few pounds. These drugs are a bitch on my weight. I'm in such crappy shape. They never gave us any time to exercise. Not that I would have. Going to have to work on that."

"You'll have plenty of time for that," I said. "I'm sure you'll get it back in control. I'm just happy to see you. Mom can't wait to see you too. She's in the car."

We grabbed Henry's bag from the belt and headed outside. Heidi was leaning against the car, searching for a sign of us. For the first time that night, I noticed what she was wearing: black corduroy pants that accented her slim frame, a plaid button-down shirt, and a pretty blue jacket that came to her thighs. Her hair was in a ponytail. Her grace and her beauty were on full display that day. I was reminded yet again of how hard I had fallen for her. Dressed up to welcome home her Henry. Her eyes scanned the crowd. When she finally caught sight of us, her whole face relaxed. She smiled, the smile I fell in love with, as she walked toward us. When she reached us, she went straight to Henry, her arms outstretched, hugging him as if her life depended on it. That embrace seemed to melt away her sadness and desperation of living with Henry's illness. Henry, too, was grinning that adorable grin of his, as he held his mother in his tall frame. I was a spectator, happy to witness this long overdue reunion. None of us knew what the future held. We were just glad to be in that moment when our lives seemed intact and filled with possibilities.

The drive home was filled with nervous energy, each of us trying to feel out our new dynamics. But all that changed as soon as we walked through the door. Bodie and Bella were ecstatic to have Henry home. They jumped on him, excited to see their long-lost friend. He played with the dogs, laughing, as they jumped all over him. It was as if we had our old Henry back.

The next day was Henry's appointment to get his teeth fixed, and he asked Heidi to join him. He might as well have asked her if she wanted a million dollars. There was nothing she wanted more than to get Henry's smile back to the one she loved. I was at work when Heidi called, whispering, "Henry got his teeth fixed." I could hear her smile through the phone. She sounded like a schoolgirl who had just had her boyhood crush nod at her as they passed in the hall.

We originally planned to go to Illinois to have Thanksgiving with Heidi's parents and her brother's family. But Covid was still rampant, and my sister-in-law was immune compromised, so we decided at the last minute not to go. My brother had asked if he could use the beach house for Thanksgiving, and I had agreed. I now called him to tell him there would be four more. We were coming.

We loved Florida, so this was not a problem. We had bought the place in 1999, and the kids had grown up going on their vacations to Florida, playing in the surf, fishing off the beach, and lounging by the pool. Our part of Florida had gotten increasingly popular over the years, and many of the homes were being replaced by larger and fancier ones. And while our neighborhood had changed as well, our house remained the same, holding on to the charms of old Florida. It was our little slice of paradise. We woke to the sounds of the waves of the Gulf of Mexico crashing and birds singing. On our long walks with the dogs, we'd see deer every time.

We were going to take two cars as I had to be in place for a Zoom meeting first thing Wednesday morning, and Heidi and Kate did not want to go until later on Wednesday. I wanted to leave Tuesday around noon. Henry decided he wanted to go with me. I told him to be ready at noon as I had to go to the office that morning. We would leave right after. I was going to drive Heidi's car since I was taking a bunch of stuff, and she had a much larger car. When I got home, the car was gone. Heidi said Henry had taken it to do some food deliveries, and when I checked he was on the Westbank of New Orleans but appeared to be heading home. I didn't know he delivered on that side of the city but thought nothing of it.

He got back about 12:30, and I held my tongue about his being late. I was getting better at that. Why pick a fight if you can avoid one? This was a new thing for me. My patience, or lack thereof, was legendary. We packed the car and were off, determined to have a nice Thanksgiving with at least two of my kids. I was just happy to have Henry back and doing so well. We drove with Henry playing the music he was listening to at the time. I remember a lot of The Strokes. We chatted about everything and nothing.

It is a four-and-a-half-hour drive, and the midway point is the tunnel in Mobile, Alabama. Growing up we were always taught that if you hold your breath as you go through a tunnel, you can make a wish, and it will come true. Some tunnels are just too damn long. Some tunnels are too short, and it seems like you're cheating to get a wish so easily granted. But that tunnel in Mobile is just right. It's hard to do with no traffic. Downright impossible with traffic. A traffic jam, don't even try. Usually you can make it, though at the end you are praying for the cars to go faster, unsure how much longer you can hold your breath. The sound of a long breath out as soon as your windshield touches sky is loud. And it feels so good. I love all my kids, but I must confess that for the last ten years, as I go through various tunnels, I have had the same wish about only one of them. A healthy and happy Henry. Like when you buy a lottery ticket and, in the back of your mind, you think you might actually win. I believed that if I wished hard enough, my wish would come true. Maybe this time, after all these wishes, it might finally be working.

The four-and-a-half-hour drive flew by, and soon we were pulling up in the driveway, the dogs wide awake, ready to play. I looked at Henry who was smiling, too. Trost, Sarah, and Harper were already there. They came out to greet us and help us unpack the car. Henry was glad to see Trost, who had always been there for him when he needed it.

Our place at the beach is not big, but there was plenty of space. Henry took the back bedroom which he would share with Kate when she arrived the next day. Henry and Kate often shared a room. Even in their twenties, they would sleep in the same bed. Kate accusing Henry of hogging the covers. Henry accusing Kate of snoring. Remembering them as young kids sleeping together flooded me with emotions. Often, we would go to wake Kate up and find an empty bed. Then, we would go into Henry's room and find her snuggled in with him. She'd had a nightmare and crawled into bed with her big brother. Her protector. Her energy twin.

I had to work most of Wednesday. Henry hung out with Trost and his family. At first, he was a little embarrassed at his weight gain, but he soon put that behind him and happily settled into catching up and talking about old times. Throughout the morning, I could hear laughter coming through the wall breaking up my call, making me wish I were with them instead of working. But soon enough the call ended, and I got to visit Trost and Henry. We went for a walk on the beach with the dogs, and Henry had a blast throwing the ball into the Gulf of Mexico, smiling each time, watching the dogs leap over the waves going headfirst into the water.

Heidi and Kate arrived late that afternoon. Henry and I went out to pick up a few pizzas for dinner. Henry was a vegan, so we also got some pasta with tomato sauce. We got back to the house around 7 p.m. Everyone was hungrily waiting for us. We all ate together, then watched a movie. I don't remember which one, but I do remember the feeling of fullness. That life could be good again. Watching Henry engrossed in a movie felt right. It felt *normal.* Something that had been absent for the last six years. Normal was a word that had been kidnapped from our lives, and now it had returned to us like a long-lost friend. I looked at Heidi, and she looked back at me. Her smile said it all.

Thanksgiving morning was frantic. The kitchen overflowed with people all trying to help. So many cooks, so little getting done. Eventually Heidi tired of Henry and me "being in the way" and suggested we go out for a walk on the beach. We took the dogs. It was a crisp, sunny day in November, warm enough to wear shorts. Henry wore his Nike shorts and a Strokes t-shirt. The day grew even warmer and sunnier as I watched him laugh and play with the dogs. Watching the smile on his face and the wind blowing his hair around, as Bella and Bodie jumped on him, was like watching a favorite movie I hadn't seen in years. When Henry looked over at me and saw my big shit-eating grin, he gave me one of his own. He was free of his troubles, at least for the moment. I was happy. The two of us on the beach, Bella and Bodie playing, and a Thanksgiving feast to look forward to with family. It seemed we had a lot to be thankful for.

By the time we came back, the Thanksgiving table was set for seven with bright colored napkins and vases of pink, red, and white roses in the middle of the table. Heidi had prepared enough vegan dishes to keep Henry full. There was a big turkey roasted a solid brown and stuffed so full it looked like some bits were trying to escape. Next to the turkey were sweet potatoes, with the marshmallows browned just right. Next to it, its cousin, mashed potatoes with butter melting on top. And there were the traditional New Orleans dishes, oyster stuffing and mirlitons stuffed with crabmeat and shrimp. There were both apple and pumpkin pies, waiting for the ice cream, still hidden in the freezer. I carved the turkey and waited for everyone to plate up and sit down. I raised the first toast. Overcome by the proximity of my family, and the lack of chaos and drama, I struggled to keep my composure. Looking at Henry, then Heidi, I just raised my glass and said how grateful I was to be surrounded by family. Then the feast began. No one spoke. All you could hear was the sound of silverware hitting plates and food being demolished. After dinner, as usual, I fell asleep in front of the TV in a food-induced coma to the sounds of Troy Aikman announcing a game between Dallas and Washington.

The next day, Henry and I decided we would try to play some tennis. We had two choices of which courts to play. One close, the other a little farther away. I wasn't sure how long Henry would last, so I picked the closer courts. Getting there, we saw that the courts were behind a locked gate. As we didn't have the code, this was a problem. The courts were directly behind a workout room and an office. I walked around to the front of the office to see if I could find anyone to help. No one was around. When I got back, Henry was still waiting patiently by the gate where I had left him.

"Well?" Henry asked, bouncing a ball on his racquet.

"I think we're out of luck. Want to go to Watercolor and just get a court for an hour?"

"Not really," Henry said, "We're already here. Let's not give up so easily. I bet I can get the code."

Then, he walked back in the direction I had just come from. After about ten minutes, I started to get impatient. I was just about to go looking for him when he popped around the corner with that big shit-eating grin on his face.

"Got it," he said, as he bent down to pick up his racquet. "Try 2314."

It worked.

"How did you get it?" I asked, incredulous.

"There was a girl working out in the gym," Henry said, pushing the gate open. "I charmed it out of her."

This was classic Henry. He had always had a way with people, and, when he wanted, he could turn it on like a faucet.

We started hitting. Nothing too strenuous, just warming up. After a few minutes, we decided to play games to eleven, a favorite of ours. As Henry was growing up, we would play points without serving and first one to eleven won. That was usually Henry. By the time he was fifteen, he could tear me apart on a tennis court. I'm a good tennis player. I played in college and still play competitively. While I can hold my own against most players, Henry was in a whole other league. There was no shot in my repertoire that could hurt him. I was too old and slow, and my strokes too soft to hit a ball that would cause him pain. As soon as he figured that out, my time was over. By age fifteen, he had learned to just hit high, heavy, topspin balls to my backhand and wait. His ball would land deep in the court and bounce like it was propelled by a rocket. If I could get my racquet on the ball at all, a major accomplishment in itself, I could do nothing more than return it weakly, the ball sitting there, waiting to be carved up. Henry would get to the ball casually and hit a forehand so hard that I'd think the cover might come off. All one hundred pounds of him would be launched at the ball, both of his feet off the ground, his racquet whirling like the blades of a helicopter. Then, the point was over. He rarely missed those shots, and I would never win again. I'm a very competitive guy, and I was not happy with this situation. But as his dad, I was proud. I never *let* him win. He just took it from me like a bully taking a kid's lunch money. But six months at a treatment center, and the weight gain had taken its toll. We played a few games of eleven, and I won all of them.

"Boy, I'm in pretty bad shape when I lose to you," Henry said, half laughing, half annoyed.

"Yep. Going to need to get back in shape. Can't be losing to your old man," I replied, half laughing, half proud of myself.

Then, he smiled at me and hit another ball. I smiled back and returned it, content to be back on the court with my favorite hitting partner.

We headed back to the house. There were a ton of leftovers to eat and some college football to watch. I pulled out the turkey and sweet potatoes from the fridge and made myself a plate. Henry had some potatoes and some fruit, then went to his room to chill. I sat down for some more football, content with how the day had gone. It had been many years since Henry and I had had fun on a tennis court, or anywhere for that matter. I was sinking deeper into my stupor when Trost announced he was leaving. It turned out he had arrived in his camper van and was going to spend a little alone time camping. I got up and walked him to his van.

"Henry seems to be doing well," he said.

"Fingers crossed," I replied.

We said our goodbyes and off he went. That night it was Sarah and Harper plus the four of us. We ate more leftovers and watched some television. Sarah and Harper left early the next morning. We started cleaning the house and were done around lunchtime. After finishing off the leftovers, we hit the road. I took the dogs and Henry rode with Heidi and Kate. That Sunday, we were back at home, lounging around watching TV when we got a call from Sarah. Trost had tested positive for Covid. She and Harper were negative. This was back in 2020 and getting such a call was no fun. The quarantine guidelines required you to remain isolated for at least five days, before you could even get tested. If you tested negative, you were released. If not, your confinement continued. While my house was not a bad place to be sheltered, no one wanted to be confined. Especially Henry, who didn't even believe Covid-19 was a disease. "Covid's not even real," was a refrain we heard many times.

To kill time, Heidi and Henry decided they wanted to play Scrabble and asked if I wanted to play. For some unknown reason, I agreed. Henry was dressed in a blue t- shirt and his favorite grey sweatpants. He was back to his old pre-illness self, being generous, allowing us to have some much-needed family time. While I was grateful, unfortunately the activity he was enjoying was Scrabble. I have never been a great Scrabble player. Scrabble is not a game for an impatient person. Everyone takes *way* too much time thinking. The game moves at a glacial pace. No one likes constantly hearing, "Are you ready yet? How much longer do you need?" Losing just makes it worse. Heidi has always been good at it, and Henry was a natural. Watching Henry and Heidi smiling as they sorted their letters like they were prizes only irritated me. Especially when my letters sucked, and I had no chance of winning. From the first seven tiles I extracted from the bag, it was clear I was in trouble. Their smirks indicated they were not. My mood continued to darken as my thumping became clearer. The score was counted, and Henry emerged the victor. I hated losing, even to my son.

My constant bickering annoyed everyone. They had both had enough, and I was not invited to play in the next round. It did allow me to take a step back and watch Heidi playing with Henry. The light in her eyes brought light to mine. The banter between them as they pondered their next move was fun to watch, like a beautiful dance. It looked so peaceful and loving, like the love I felt when I watched my kids sleeping. Those two were having so much fun they didn't even notice me. It had been a while since I'd seen them have any fun together. A game of Scrabble had seemed unimaginable six months ago. I walked away, listening to them laughing and making fun of me. Maybe things were getting back to normal. Maybe the six-month stay had done what we had hoped. Maybe we could be the family Heidi and I had always thought we could be. Maybe.

chapter 33

HOUSE CALL

It was Tuesday morning December 1, and Heidi drove Henry to get his monthly shot of Abilify, the anti-psychotic he was on. And to me, a miracle drug. She returned home with him while I was upstairs working. Around noon I was getting hungry and came downstairs to grab a bite. I saw Heidi in the kitchen. "Where's Henry?" I asked.

"He took Kate's car and went for a run by the river in the French Quarter. He asked if you were home, but I thought you were at the office. He should be back soon."

It seemed weird to me that Henry would go running in the Quarter when Audubon Park was only half a mile away. I checked his location on my phone. He was back on the Westbank in the same vicinity he had been to a week ago. This made no sense to me, so I checked what was near where his little blue dot was flashing. Gretna Gun Works. Not good.

A week before Henry had punched me, back in May, when he was severely manic, he had posted to Instagram a picture of himself at a gun store. Heidi saw it and called me in a panic. I started dialing gun stores. I could see where he was, so I called the closest gun store and sure enough he had been there. I told them he had bipolar disorder and to not sell him a gun. They assured me that his unwell mental state had been obvious. They had not sold him a gun. I then called every gun store that I could in the New Orleans area—there were a lot of them—and I told them the same thing. At that time all assured me that they would not sell him one. Including Gretna Gun works.

That morning, hardly comprehending the lie we had been told but realizing the truth of his location, I called Gretna Gun Works. After a long time on hold, someone finally picked up. I explained to them Henry's situation and pleaded with them not to sell him a gun. The woman said that they were busy, and someone would call me back. She quickly hung up on me. Stunning, I thought, gun sales before everything. At this point Heidi was frantic. I was not as worried and tried to calm her down. I had given Gretna Gun Works his name. Surely, they wouldn't sell him a gun. I called his cell but no answer. I called five more times before giving up, as if my repeated calls would get him to answer. I was growing concerned, though at this point there was nothing I could do. I went back upstairs to try to finish my work. Work, however, proved impossible. All I could think about was Henry and where he was. Heidi couldn't wait and, without telling me, immediately got in her car and drove off looking for him.

I had been upstairs for about fifteen minutes when Kate came up to tell me the police were on the front porch. As I walked down the stairs, my first thought was that Henry had been arrested again. How nice of them to make a house call.

Yet, in the back of my mind, of course, I knew that cops didn't make house calls to tell you your son has been arrested. I got to the front door to see two plain clothes police officers dressed in black pants and black polo shirts standing there. One was at the door, and the other was a couple of steps back, looking down as if to avoid any eye contact. They didn't have to say anything. I knew. I just knew that my dear Henry, my sweet boy, was gone. I could see it in their faces. Delivering news like this is a hard job. I'm sure they wanted to be there about as much as I wanted them there. "Mr. Friedler, I'm sorry to say this. Henry Friedler was found deceased in his car at 11:30 this morning."

I once heard someone say, "It is one thing to imagine being chased by a bear. It is an entirely different thing actually being chased by a bear." And the bear had caught my son. And while I always knew this day might come, I was woefully unprepared for its arrival. The ground beneath me fell away. It became hard to breathe. A gut punch that knocks you out. The world as you knew it was over. The emptiness felt like a black hole impossible to fill. I could see that the officers were talking, their mouths moving, but I didn't hear any of it. I could feel the blood draining from my face. My body was being pulled down by a heavy gravity that I couldn't fight. The darkness engulfed me. I didn't even know where I was. The only thing I felt was the embrace of despair, and it would not let go. My legs gave out, and I had to sit down. This was a terrible dream, yet I was awake. My thoughts quickly darkened. I had called the cell phone of my dead son. Had it been next to his body, ringing and ringing? Did his soul hear it, unable to answer? My brain was filled with crazy thoughts yet no thoughts at all. I was numb. The police were still on our porch, still talking, and it took me a second to hear the words.

"He bought a gun, went right to his car, and shot himself. I know this is hard. We are both sorry for your loss. His body will be released soon, as given what we found we do not think an autopsy is necessary. Do you have any questions for us?"

Yes. I have a lot of questions. Why? Why now? Why did he do it? He was doing so well. We were so hopeful. Instead, I said, "No. Not really." They said they would be in touch with more details soon and left.

Kate was in our entrance hall, sitting on a chair crying. She looked like a broken doll. Her energy twin was gone. I tried to console her. She was inconsolable. But I continued to hold her. I was still in shock. In the back of all our minds, we knew that a diagnosis of bipolar often does not end well. While many can get through life in some fashion—some do fine, others not so much—many lives end in suicide. That was always the phone call we were dreading. Now, it was our reality. Heidi needed to know. I was glad that it would be me telling her. I was devastated that it would be me telling her. First, I needed her home. I needed to be able to hold her when I told her, and she needed to get back home. I made the call.

"Heidi, you need to come home."

"Why? I need to find Henry." Her voice grew more desperate with each word.

"You just need to come home. We can talk when you get home."

Now, she was crying. "Why? What happened to him? Where is he? What is going on? Please tell me." she begged.

What could I say? She knew just like I had, but I needed her home. "Just come home."

It took twenty minutes for Heidi to get home. It seemed like twenty hours. I was wandering my house with no intentions at all. Only moving felt right. As if I were to quit moving, I would fall apart. I heard Heidi's car pull up. She came through the front door with red eyes that were pleading with me not to tell her what she already knew. She took one look at me and broke down. She was wild-eyed and gushing tears. She looked at me and kept saying, "No. No. No. It can't be. No." I had not yet opened my mouth, but the look on my face and the look on Kate's face said everything. I grabbed her and literally held her up as she sank down into the darkness I knew all too well. "My baby. My poor baby. Why? Why? No. No." I held her for what seemed like ten minutes. It was probably less. I tried to hold her and protect her, but I was way too late. Her worst nightmare had come true. I slowly put her on the ground then got on the floor myself and hugged her some more, as if I could hug the sadness out of her. If I held her long enough, all of this would go away. I felt bad for Kate who was also in pain. Her brother was gone, and her loss was obvious. She just kept crying and shaking her head. But I was focused on Heidi and holding her. She just kept crying, and I felt so small and helpless next to this absolute and pure grief.

While Heidi and Kate were in the throes of despair, I realized there was a lot to do. This was a weird thought in the grip of such pain. I needed something to do to keep me from thinking about the pain. Why and how I got it together I can't say. But I knew I had to make three phone calls. First, I had to call Patti in Chicago.

"Patti, I have bad news."

"What? What happened?" By the way she asked, you knew she knew.

"Henry killed himself about an hour ago."

Silence. Nothing. Then crying. Not being able to hold Patti left a hole in my heart. It made me feel like a spectator in a game that was my life. I stayed on the phone with her as she cried, whispering to her that it would be alright. Lying to her. It was far from alright, and she knew it. There was nothing I could say other than come home. She was home the next day.

The next two calls were to his grandparents. I called Heidi's parents first. I dialed Chuck, somehow knowing he would be with Lori. I was right. They were in the car going somewhere. As I was numb to everything, there was no preamble. "Chuck, Henry killed himself. We just found out." "What?" This kind of news was not what he was expecting. In the background I could hear Lori asking, "What? What is going on?" Then, Chuck telling her and her saying, "Oh my god, no. Oh my god." He was clearly blindsided and was muttering to me something I could not make out. "We will check the flights. We will probably be down tomorrow. Poor Heidi. Is she there? Can we talk to her?"

"Now is not a great time," I said. "She's really bad. If you want, you can try her cell. I'll tell her you're coming. Let me know the flight number, and I'll arrange to have someone get you. Can you tell Chip and Jenny."

My next call was to Pam, my stepmom and Henry's grand-mother on my side. Pam and Dad had always been close to the kids, and, while Dad was dead, Pam was still their grand-mother, their Mimi. They all loved her.

"Pam, Henry is dead. He killed himself." "What? Are you kidding?" "No. He is dead." Silence. She was taking a while to gather her composure.

"Will you call Carey and Trost and tell them?"

"Of course," she said. "Is there anything else I can do. I am so sorry. I don't know what to say."

Of course not. Who does? There is nothing to say. Our son was dead, and that was it. No amount of wishing could make it different. Believe me, I tried.

chapter 34

HENRY

December 5, 2020, was a beautiful day in New Orleans. The weather was brisk but not cold, and the sun was out. And although the sky was blue, the mood was impossibly grey. As I looked out over the crowd seated on white chairs on the neutral ground outside our house, there were many familiar faces. There were friends from all over the country, from every point in our lives. They were there to honor Henry. My poor brave Henry who had killed himself four days earlier. He was twenty-seven when he died. The police report would say that he died of a self-inflicted gunshot wound, but the real culprit was an insidious disease. As we gathered that day, our world had fallen apart. But the sight of so many friends there to honor our son buoyed our flagging spirits.

We were still in the throes of Covid. The vaccine would not be out for another month, and not many were willing to have services of any kind. No weddings, no birthday parties, and no funerals. But it was inconceivable to Heidi and me that we could not honor Henry, so thanks to two great friends, Debbie Marx and Vicky Sperling, we set up chairs in front of our house, got a microphone, and had a service. Henry would have loved it, I think. A boy who often felt invisible in life and now all too visible in death. He would have loved seeing all his friends, many of whom had long given up on him. I don't blame them. Bipolar is a tough one. And Henry had been particularly manic. It was hard to be his dad, and I think it would have been next to impossible to be his friend.

The night before the service, we discussed amongst ourselves who'd give the eulogies. Kate wanted to speak. To my surprise so did Heidi. Heidi's always been brilliant and articulate, but she's a deeply private person. To want to expose her grief in front of so many people was unlike her. To open herself up in that way, especially as raw as she was, made me appreciate her even more. The world was going to get a chance to see the courageous person I was married to. The fighter no one gets to see. While I wanted to protect her, it was clear she did not need protecting.

I was even more surprised to learn that Heidi had saved the dress she wore at Ian's funeral and that she planned on wearing it again at Henry's. I had no idea she'd saved that dress, that she had held on to this trace of Ian after all of these years. And that she had done so, in silence, not even sharing it with me. Keeping it her secret, as if the dress had the power to protect her from anything bad happening again. But it hadn't worked. And she would wear it again.

As usual, I wanted the last word. But Heidi insisted that the last words be hers. This beautiful woman, so broken by the loss of her son, showed a strength few get to see. Heidi is the rock of our family. She had done all she could to help Henry in his battle. She had done her best to will Henry into getting better. But the disease won. She was broken in ways that are impossible to describe. But she wanted the world to see a fuller picture of Henry. She wanted the world to know that this illness didn't define him, that he was a sweet caring boy, a gifted artist, a young man who was much greater than his disease. Heidi wanted them to know he was curious about the world and relentless in his pursuits. He was everything you would want in a son. She wanted to tell his truth to the world. She wanted Henry's beauty to be the final thought at her son's memorial. I'm not sure I have ever loved her more than I did that day.

Looking out over a sea of faces of those who loved Henry and who loved us, I was filled with a wave of joy. I was still devastated over our loss, so this emotion is hard to explain. I think the adrenaline rush of speaking about Henry to friends made my loss just a little easier to bear. Before we all went outside to begin the service, we were wracked with grief. I think we were all in tears or close to it. Stephen Godchaux, our close friend who loved Henry very much and had been his Los Angeles guardian, reminded us that we needed to try to get through our speeches as the service was about Henry and not about us. So, as only I can do, I made it a competition. The one who cried the most lost. For those wondering, that would be Kate. Her energy twin was gone. She took the loss very hard, but she was brave enough to share with the crowd her love for her brother. She cried. The crowd cried. I cried. Kate was spectacular.

Heidi's talk was heartbreaking. She talked about Henry and his journey. All she wanted for Henry was a carefree and happy life. She was heartbroken over her loss and grief-stricken about all the struggles he had had to endure, which she shared with the crowd. Her bravery, while not surprising to me, was powerful for others to witness. Her telling of Henry's fight with his illness was gut-wrenching to hear. Mental illness is a mysterious beast, one with so many questions and so few answers. It is still a disease that comes with terrible shame, which makes coping with it even more difficult. A mental illness diagnosis doesn't bring care packages and casseroles. No one wants to be near it. Sympathy and empathy for the sufferer are nearly impossible to find. Henry had to fight his battle alone, as did our whole family. I challenge anyone to visit a cancer wing of a hospital and then a mental health wing—you'll understand what I'm saying. Heidi bringing to light Henry's struggles was long overdue and necessary. She also urged people to be more empathetic to those who suffer from mental illness and to those who care for them. She closed the services with forbearance and grace and was right about being the last to speak. Having to follow her would have been unimaginable.

Since we were in the middle of the pandemic, we weren't able to receive all the love and hugs that people wanted to give us. We waved to people as this long sad line of friends and family walked in front of us. The crowd dispersed, and we went back inside, alone with just our family and the friends who had traveled to New Orleans to be with us.

Words have meaning, of course. After Henry's death, people used words to try to give us comfort. We would hear "sorry for your loss," and, while it was a "loss," it trivialized what we were experiencing. I appreciated their well-intentioned words, but they didn't work. "Loss" is just an easier way to say that Henry was dead. Our boy was not lost. We knew exactly where he was. Dead. Even the word hurts. To make death seem more manageable, we often say our loved one *has died*, as if it were in the past, the person stacked up on a shelf and put away. We also hear that our loved one *has passed*. To me this connotes a tranquility to death that didn't exist in a case like Henry's. We rarely say our loved one *is* dead. This present tense stays with us. A brutal finality. It's not surprising that we want to soften the blow of death by using other words. Yet, who are those soft words for? Not the loved ones left behind. No amount of "softness" could erase the pain we felt. There are no words that could bring us comfort. I wanted Henry alive, and short of that there was nothing anyone could do for me. And there were no words that would help. A touch, perhaps. A hug, definitely. Just being there, sitting with me in my misery, absolutely. Words just fell short.

Our boy is dead. I recognize this sounds harsh. It is. Death is harsh, especially a child's death. It's not the way the world is supposed to work. A child's death seems unfair and unnatural. Yet, that was our truth. But you hold on to whatever you can, even if it's a dress. Ian was only three months. Henry was twenty-seven. Ian died of natural causes while Henry killed himself. Each death is separate and distinct, connected only by the commonality of heartbreak and despair. But this time it was our beloved Henry, and, while the "loss" is alike, this one felt far worse. Reality began to set in. The mourning was just beginning, and, while I knew, because of Ian, each year would get a little easier, it was hard to make myself believe it. My son was gone, and the hole in our hearts seemed impossible to fill.

chapter 35

TUNNELS

For the first week, everyone tries to be there for you. We ate
well for a week or so, with friends bringing dinner to our house
every evening. As this was New Orleans, the food was quite
good. Vicky was in charge. She would call us every day and let
us know who was cooking for us that night. Lamb chops one
night, crawfish étouffée the next. A redfish dish that melted in
your mouth. If there is such a thing as comfort food, this was
it. Yet it brought no comfort.

And even that eventually ended. Patti went back to Chicago
after about a week. Kate returned to her life, though she came
over all the time. She needed to be with those who understood.

I suspect it was hard for friends to visit our house. We
were engulfed in a sadness that was palpable and all-con-
suming. Only the brave would venture over. Our closest
friends did what they could. But our world had gone dark,
and no light could get through. I could be anywhere in the
house and still hear Heidi crying uncontrollably. It was a pri-
mal sound, somewhere between screaming and crying. Soul
crushing wails. I would find her and hold her until she had
nothing left. I learned that just being there and letting her
be sad was all I could do. And that was hard. I had spent the

last ten years trying to live with Heidi's sadness, to be comfortable near it and with it. Now, I was getting a master class in despair and felt I was failing. Her complete sadness made me feel that I was not being sad enough. Why was Heidi so devastated, and I could go on? Despite my ongoing grief, I eventually returned to my normal routine, going to work every day and dealing with clients. What was wrong with me? I tried to look back at our path from the misery that Ian's death had created. All I could remember was that I could not remember. I certainly couldn't remember pain like this. Yet, that pain *had* existed, and that pain *had* waned. I knew that our journey would be long and awful. I also knew that it would be measured in inches, not feet.

The next few months passed quickly and slowly at the same time. I was there but not really, like I was living in a fog I couldn't see out of. I only remember the cloud of darkness we were living under. Like Pigpen and his cloud of dust, it followed us everywhere we went.

During the months that followed, there were two moments that did help, and both involved friends of Henry. Steve, Henry's friend who five years earlier had written me that harsh letter telling me how I should handle Henry after he took the mescalin, was living out of town and, therefore, had been unable to come to the memorial. After Henry's death he wrote to me. *That* letter I did save. It showed how much he had loved our Henry. The letter was beautiful and heartbreaking. To this day, I reread it and cry. A few months after Henry died,

Steve was in town and texted me asking if he could come by to see Heidi and me. What bravery. Not only was he willing to come into this house of darkness, he was coming after having told me, in all his youthful audacity, I did not truly know my son. He came over on a Saturday, and we sat in our library, the cozy room we refer to as the Red Room, with its red rug, red curtains, grey couch, and two red chairs backed by over-flowing bookshelves. Heidi, Steve, and I sat in that room and talked about Henry for nearly three hours. It was emotional in all the right ways, and heartbreaking in all the right ways. Henry came alive again in Steve's words and generous tone. That gift stayed with us a long time, and I will always cherish the time Steve gave us.

Later that summer Henry's friend Josh came to visit. Josh and Henry had been friends since preschool at Uptown Montessori. During his illness Henry had been particularly mean to Josh in the same way he had been mean to us. He was harshest on the ones he loved the most. Josh had stayed away from Henry and at the service was uncontrollably sad. He cried for the friend he had lost a second time. As much pain as we were in, it was comforting seeing someone else so broken by Henry's death, someone who missed him as much as we did. Six months later I reached out to Josh asking if he wanted one of Henry's sport coats. I really just wanted another connection to my son, and seeing Josh heartbroken at Henry's memorial had stayed with me. Josh came over on a Sunday and stayed for an hour. He cried. We cried. We told stories about Henry, reviving him again, at least for that hour. Those two acts of kindness continue to nourish us.

Before we knew it, summer was on us like a fast car barreling down the road, and Watervale was around the next turn. We had a lot of Watervale friends who wanted to memorialize Henry, so we agreed to have a service our first Sunday there. Heidi was weighed down by the burden of it all. I could tell the thought of another memorial was taking a toll on her. I tried to convince her that this would be cathartic and that our friends wanted to be there for us. None of us really wanted to relive this. Yet, I felt we owed it to our friends. And that's crazy, of course. Why did I feel the need to comfort others? Their son had not died, mine had. Why was I worried about their feelings? Yet, that's what you are often forced to do: to live with that uncomfortable silence between people who don't know what to say. To rescue them from the darkness that we live in every day.

So instead of looking forward to Watervale, Heidi was dreading it. She didn't want to have the memorial. But in the blink of an eye, we were at Watervale, and it was Sunday morning. After breakfast, we all gathered by the tennis courts. The sky was azure blue, not a cloud in it. It was seventy-five degrees with no humidity, the kind of day that reminds us why we love Watervale so much. There were around thirty people in attendance. Jenny, who runs Watervale, was there, as well as some other Watervale staff who knew us and Henry. There were the friends with whom we had spent this week for the last twenty years in a row, watching our children grow up together since they were babies. I could see Heidi starting to tear up with the love and warmth she was getting from this group, a group we are with for only one week a year who nevertheless feel like best friends. Kate, Heidi, and I all spoke. There was not a dry set of eyes that morning. The love we felt was warm and comforting, like sitting by a fire in the dead of winter. Afterwards, Heidi and I took a walk. She was relieved it was over and felt better that we had done it. She was buoyed by the fact that so many people cared. For the moment life was bearable.

The next day after breakfast, Jenny asked if she could come by our cottage. An hour later she walked up, carrying a large stone with Henry's name inscribed on it. She explained it was a lake stone indigenous to the area. She told us it was ours to do what we wanted with it. We were so touched we all started to cry, Jenny included. We talked amongst ourselves and agreed that the best place for it was in the garden next to the tennis court, in a little spot surrounded by wildflowers. Heidi and I took it over and placed it in the garden with some of Henry's ashes. We held hands and sat in silence, staring at his name. It was quiet and still. We looked at each other. A calm came over us, and for a second, we could feel him with us. It was nice to know that for the rest of time Henry's name would be sitting next to the courts he loved so much.

That first Thanksgiving after Henry's death was a tough one. My favorite holiday was quickly turning into my least favorite. I can't envision a Thanksgiving when Henry will not be my first thought.

I have a client who has a family retreat on the Wednesday before Thanksgiving in Sea Island, Georgia, and I wanted to be at that meeting. Heidi agreed to have Thanksgiving in Florida to accommodate me. It's only a six-hour drive to Sea Island from Santa Rosa Beach, and I didn't want to deal with airports on the Wednesday before Thanksgiving. So, I drove alone to Florida the Friday before, giving me a few days at the beach before my drive to Sea Island. As I approached the Mobile tunnel, my thoughts turned to Henry, as they do every time I go through a tunnel. This would be my first time driving through it since Henry's death. My wish would have to change. I held my breath unable to come up with another one. What else mattered? My son was dead, and I felt I had nothing left to wish for. Yet, I continued to hold my breath out of respect for Henry. There was traffic, and it was hard. I needed to breathe but refused to quit. Do it for Henry, I kept saying. When I reached the end, I exhaled loudly, sucking in breaths like they were valuable. At that moment I realized that Henry's tunnel had been too long for him. He hadn't been able to make it. I drove the rest of the way with watery eyes, feeling guilty that my wishes had not worked.

I spent a few days at the beach alone before heading to Sea Island for my meeting. Still feeling a little disoriented, I needed this time to regroup and reframe my thoughts. Long walks on the beach with the dogs helped. Heidi and Kate arrived on

Monday. That helped, as well. By Tuesday I was ready for the drive to Sea Island to meet with my clients the next day.

This family is one of the nicest and sweetest families I know. There are three generations at the meeting, twenty people seated around a large, circular conference table. At the end of every meeting, they do a roll call where each person in attendance lets everyone else know what is going on with them—my favorite part of the meeting. This was my first meeting after Henry's death. Patti had flown in that Wednesday, so we could have Thanksgiving as a family. Our new family of four. That was something I was not sure I would ever get used to. I knew that Heidi was going to have a tough time. Her first without Henry. Coming back to Florida, the place where she last spent time with Henry, was going to make it even tougher. I knew I had to hurry back to be with Heidi. This family had been incredibly supportive of me and had all come up to me at the start of the meeting to express their condolences. Since I knew I had to get back, I went first. With a crackle in my throat, I let them know how much their family meant to me. I told them that I had to leave and get back to Heidi. They understood, and I left for my six-hour drive back.

It was a tough six hours. All my thoughts went to Henry. I thought back to the last time we played tennis. I thought back to that little kid with the great smile. The kind of smile that let you know he knew he was onto something. That he was into everything. The kid who was curious about *everything*. The kid who would sleep with his DK books. The kid who was a terror on the soccer fields, running and laughing with his teammates. The kid who would build forts with his friends on the third floor of our house. Then the kid who was overwhelmed by his demons. The kid who had to fight a disease without much help. The warrior who fought as best as he could and decided he could fight no more. I thought of the loneliness of his last moments, sitting in that car. It hurt so much to think how alone he must have felt.

When you have a child who kills himself, it is natural to wonder why. This is a fool's errand, of course. There's no way to get in their head. A friend wrote me something that has stayed with me all these years. He wrote, "But in another way, we are all strangers to what really boils deep inside others—even those closest to us." As I drove back to Florida, I was trying to figure out why. But I had been doing it through *my* filter, which I knew by now was never going to work. In coming to grips with Henry's ending, I decided to choose what I believed.

I believe he knew he was loved.

I believe he was tired of his fight.

I believe he believed he was doing the right thing.

I believe he believed he was doing the loving thing.

It was not what I would have chosen. It wasn't my choice. It was Henry's. We live on and know that the world will be a little less bright and a lot less interesting without him in it. But Henry is at peace. Finally.

epilogue

In June of 2022, hope resurfaced. Two days before our annual trip to Watervale, Patti's boyfriend, Ben, called to tell us he was going to ask Patti to marry him during our week at Watervale and wanted our blessing. Ben asked us to keep it a secret until he proposed. While our excitement was hard to hide, especially from Kate, Heidi and I would do a little dance every time we were alone. A little jig with small movements but big smiles.

The next Monday, in a private moment, Ben asked Patti. For the first time, I could see light at the end of our tunnel. The chance finally to exhale. The cherry on top, in a part of America known for its cherries, was that Patti wanted to get married at Watervale. This special place of ours was soon to get even more special. The next year flew by. Heidi was overwhelmed with planning a wedding, but I would still hear her crying throughout the house. She missed Henry. Of course she did. We all did. He had died only two years earlier. Yet, she persevered with purpose, as she always has. The tranquility of Watervale was going to complement her vision of what Patti's wedding could be.

Before we knew it, September 2023 was upon us. It had been a stressful year for Heidi, and I was worried that she wouldn't be able to enjoy the moment. Sons escort their mothers down the aisle at weddings, and Heidi was deeply sad that this tradition was never going to happen. While looking forward to her daughter's wedding, she was still buried deep in grief.

On September 4, 2023, as we made the drive from Chicago to Watervale hauling a trailer full of wedding supplies, I was concerned. This all changed as we drove into Watervale. Descending the last hill and turning on to Watervale Road, I could see Heidi's posture straighten. Her face relaxed. The weather was cold and rainy, but Heidi was warm and sunny. And sure enough, over the next few days, the weather caught up to Heidi's brightening mood. By Friday afternoon, Watervale was filled with our friends and family and sun.

Friday night was our welcome dinner, a traditional Watervale barbecue. Seeing many of our favorite people in our favorite place made a beautiful late summer afternoon even more beautiful. We scheduled dinner on the early side, so we could move the party down to the beach for sunset. Watervale always has spectacular sunsets, with Lake Michigan swallowing the sun. This one might have been the best. As the bright orange circle sank below the blue horizon of Lake Michigan, Heidi and I held hands. For the first time in a long time, Henry came up, and we smiled.

The next morning, we woke to clear blue skies. It was sixty-eight degrees. The kind of weather that makes Watervale *Watervale*. Heidi and I took about forty people on our Baldy hike. Walking through the woods, running down Baldy, Heidi was smiling and laughing as she showed her girlfriends the

Watervale she loved. The word "perfect" was invented for a moment like this.

And then the wedding was upon us. Patti on my arm, with our friends and family seated on the deck overlooking Lower Lake Herring, is as close to heaven as I can imagine. Looking that day at Patti, a thirty-three-year-old woman in her wedding dress about to meet the love of her life at the altar, was life-changing. I wish I could have stayed in that moment forever. Seeing my entire family so happy brought me a level of contentment I forgot existed. While life can be unfair, it also gives you gifts like these. The joy of the moment sucked all the oxygen away from sadness. It had happened after Ian's death when Patti was born. But I had forgotten. And that lesson had been lost. On this day it was re-learned. Watching Ben and Patti getting married, with Kate by her side and Heidi by mine, made me realize what I had instead of what I was missing. And I had a lot.

In typical New Orleans fashion, we second-lined over to the reception, Patti and Ben leading the way, their white and black umbrellas held high in the air and the brass band playing "When The Saints Go Marching In." Our family experienced a joy unimaginable three years earlier. Our friends kept commenting on how much we deserved a night like this. A weekend like this. If it was deserved, I'm not sure. But I do know we took it.

Our father-daughter dance was to "You Can't Always Get What You Want" by the Rolling Stones, a song that had particular meaning to our family. And yes, we ached for Henry. His absence, a notable hole in our celebration. And yes, I wanted desperately to see him become the person I knew him to be. But on this particular night, looking at Patti so happy, looking at Kate and Heidi glowing, surrounded by our friends and family, I realized that we had a future. We had made it through our tunnel and could finally breathe again. And it felt good.

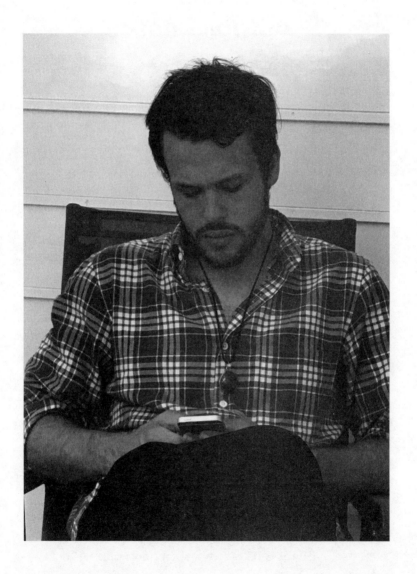

author's note

There were no real source materials for this book. It was all done from memory and notes taken by Heidi during the many years of Henry's illness. I have changed a few names and places to protect people's privacy. The conversations I recreate are as I remember them, though they should not be taken word-for-word. They do recreate both the feeling and meaning of what was said. As with all memories they can fade but to the best of my ability everything in this story takes place as written. Each of us has our own version of the truth. This is mine.

There are many great mental health resources. Here are a few.

Contact your local NAMI Affiliate www.nami.org to find the affiliate closest to you for individual mental help guidance, services and programs for yourself or as a loved one.

Contact SAMHSA National Helpline, a free, confidential, 24/7, 365-day-a-year referral and information Service at 1-800-662 HELP (4357)

In New Orleans contact CALM at 504-988-0301 or www.calmnola.org

acknowledgements

This was a tough book to write, and I have many people to thank. First and foremost, would be Heidi who put up with me asking question after question when answering them was the last thing she wanted to do. I kept asking and she kept handling me as only she knows how. My love for her is endless.

I had many readers along the way but two jumped out and need special acknowledgment. Sassy Kohlmeyer was there from the beginning. We took many a walk around Audubon Park and her patience and many reads were beyond helpful. It takes a real friend to say, "you can do better." She is a real friend. Stephen Godchaux is the second. Not only was he a dear friend to Henry, he has been a lifelong friend of mine. He took time out of his very busy day to help me edit every single word. We spent the better part of three months working on making this book the best it could be, and it would not exist without Stephen's help and patience.

I also need to thank a handful of other people who read this at least once and whose insights made it better. Adam Hawf, Charlie Crosby, Randy Fertel, Karen Taggert, Rachel Butler, Andrew Sperling and Stephen Phillipson, all gave me valuable feedback that helped make this a better book. A special shoutout to Merritt Lane who enabled me to get this book distributed in a way that people could find it. Also, a shout out to Micheal Lewis, Robbie Vitrano, Debbie Marx, Sam Burkhardt. TJ Locke, Serena Chaudry, Dr. Ashley Weiss, Jack Weiss, Tom Lowenburg of Octavia Books and Bryan Beasley of Sundog Books.

There were many people on Team Tripp in working on the book. My editors Nayana Abeysinghe who helped birth the book and Kristen Sanders who helped deliver it. Carrie Chappell gave it a final review and added some well-placed edits. My design team led by Pat McGuinness and the team at Trumpet. And my PR team led by Steve O'Keefe.

Finally, to all my clients and my fellow members of the FreeGulliver team for putting up with me when I was writing. I appreciate you all.